D1269305

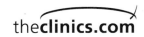

PHYSICAL MEDICINE AND REHABILITATION CLINICS OF NORTH AMERICA

New Advances in Prosthetics and Orthotics

GUEST EDITOR
Mark H. Bussell, MD, CPO

CONSULTING EDITOR
George H. Kraft, MD, MS

February 2006 • Volume 17 • Number 1

SAUNDERS

An Imprint of Elsevier, Inc.
PHILADELPHIA   LONDON   TORONTO   MONTREAL   SYDNEY   TOKYO

W.B. SAUNDERS COMPANY
A Division of Elsevier Inc.

1600 John F. Kennedy Blvd. • Suite 1800 • Philadelphia, Pennsylvania 19103

http://www.theclinics.com

PHYSICAL MEDICINE AND REHABILITATION	Volume 17, Number 1
CLINICS OF NORTH AMERICA	ISSN 1047-9651
February 2006	ISBN 1-4160-3588-5
Editor: Debora Dellapena	

Copyright © 2006 Elsevier Inc. All rights reserved. No part of this publication may be reproduced or transmitted in any form or by any means, electronic or mechanical, including photocopy, recording, or any information storage and retrieval system, without written permission from the publisher.

Single photocopies of single articles may be made for personal use as allowed by national copyright laws. Permission of the publisher and payment of a fee is required for all other photocopying, including multiple or systematic copying, copying for advertising or promotional purposes, resale, and all forms of document delivery. Special rates are available for educational institutions that wish to make photocopies for non-profit educational classroom use. Permissions may be sought directly from Elsevier's Rights Department in Philadelphia, PA, USA: phone: (+1) 215 239 3804, fax: (+1) 215 239 3805, e-mail: healthpermissions@elsevier.com. Requests may also be completed on-line via the Elsevier homepage (http://www.elsevier.com/locate/permissions). In the USA, users may clear permissions and make payments through the Copyright Clearance Center, Inc., 222 Rosewood Drive, Danvers, MA 01923, USA; phone: (978) 750-8400, fax: (978) 750-4744, and in the UK through the Copyright Licensing Agency Rapid Clearance Service (CLARCS), 90 Tottenham Court Road, London W1P 0LP, UK; phone: (+44) 171 436 5931; fax: (+44) 171 436 3986. Other countries may have a local reprographic rights agency for payments.

The ideas and opinions expressed in *Physical Medicine and Rehabilitation Clinics of North America* do not necessarily reflect those of the Publisher. The Publisher does not assume any responsibility for any injury and/or damage to persons or property arising out of or related to any use of the material contained in this periodical. The reader is advised to check the appropriate medical literature and the product information currently provided by the manufacturer of each drug to be administered to verify the dosage, the method and duration of administration, or contraindications. It is the responsibility of the treating physician or other health care professional, relying on independent experience and knowledge of the patient, to determine drug dosages and the best treatment for the patient. Mention of any product in this issue should not be construed as endorsement by the contributors, editors, or the Publisher of the product or manufacturers' claims.

Physical Medicine and Rehabilitation Clinics of North America (ISSN 1047-9651) is published quarterly by W.B. Saunders, 360 Park Avenue South, New York, NY 10010-1710. Months of publication are February, May, August, and November. Business and Editorial Offices: 1600 John F. Kennedy Blvd., Suite 1800, Philadelphia, PA 19103-2899. Accounting and Circulation Offices: 6277 Sea Harbor Drive, Orlando, FL 32887-4800. Periodicals postage paid at New York, NY and additional mailing offices. Subscription price per year is $160.00 (US individuals), $250.00 (US institutions), $80.00 (US students), $195.00 (Canadian individuals), $320.00 (Canadian institutions), $110.00 (Canadian students), $225.00 (foreign individuals), $320.00 (foreign institutions), and $110.00 (foreign students). Foreign air speed delivery is included in all *Clinics* subscription prices. All prices are subject to change without notice. POSTMASTER: Send address changes to *Physical Medicine and Rehabilitation Clinics of North America*, Elsevier Periodicals Customer Service, 6277 Sea Harbor Drive, Orlando, FL 32887-4800. **Customer Service: 1-800-654-2452 (US). From outside of the US, call 1-407-345-4000.**

Physical Medicine and Rehabilitation Clinics of North America is indexed in *Excerpta Medica, Index Medicus, Cinahl,* and *Cumulative Index to Nursing and Allied Health Literature.*

Printed in the United States of America.

CONSULTING EDITOR

GEORGE H. KRAFT, MD, MS, Alvord Professor of Multiple Sclerosis Research Professor, Department of Rehabilitation Medicine; Adjunct Professor of Neurology; Director, Electrodiagnostic Medicine, Western Multiple Sclerosis Center; and Co-Director, Muscular Dystrophy Clinic, The University of Washington, Seattle, Washington

GUEST EDITOR

MARK H. BUSSELL, MD, CPO, Fort Worth, Texas

CONTRIBUTORS

ROBERT A. BEDOTTO, PT, CPO, CPI, President and Chief Clinician, OrthoTherapy LLC at Bray Orthotics and Prosthetics, Westwood, New Jersey

GENE P. BERNARDONI, CO, President and Director of Clinical Services, Ballert Orthopedic of Chicago; and Lecturer, Northwestern University Medical School Prosthetic-Orthotic Center, Chicago, Illinois

DALE BERRY, CP, FAAOP, Vice-President, Clinical Operations, Hanger Orthopedic Group, Golden Valley, Minnesota

KEVIN CARROLL, MS, CP, FAAOP, Vice-President of Prosthetics, Hanger Prosthetics & Orthotics, Orlando, Florida

DONALD R. CUMMINGS, CP (LP), Department of Prosthetics, Texas Scottish Rite Hospital for Children, Dallas, Texas

ROBERT DODSON, CPO, Advanced Arm Dynamics of Texas, Irving, Texas

NANCY WILLIAMS ELFTMAN, CO, CPed, President, Hands on Foot, Inc.; President, Cosmos Extremity, Inc., La Verne, California

THOMAS M. GAVIN, CO, President and Director of Clinical Services, BioConcepts, Inc., Burr Ridge; and Research Orthotist, Musculoskeletal Biomechanics Laboratory, Veterans Administration Hospital, Hinsdale, Illinois

TIM GOLDBERG, CP, LPO, Director of Prosthetics, ProsthetiCare Fort Worth, Fort Worth, Texas

TODD KUIKEN, MD, PhD, Director, Neural Engineering Center for Artificial Limbs, Rehabilitation Institute of Chicago; and Associate Professor, Departments of Physical

Medicine Rehabilitation and Biomedical Engineering, Northwestern University, Chicago, Illinois

CHRIS LAKE, CPO, FAAOP, Advanced Arm Dynamics of Texas, Irving, Texas

MARMADUKE D. R. LOKE, CPO, President, DynamicBracingSolutions, Inc., San Diego, California

ROSS QUERRY, PhD, PT, Assistant Professor, Department of Physical Therapy, The University of Texas Southwestern Medical Center, Dallas, Texas

JOHN P. SPAETH, MS, CP, Midwest Regional Vice President, Hanger Prosthetics & Orthotics, Bethesda, Maryland

TED A. TROWER, CPO, A-S-C Orthotics & Prosthetics, Jackson, Michigan

PATRICIA WINCHESTER, PhD, PT, Professor and Chair, Department of Physical Therapy, The University of Texas Southwestern Medical Center, Dallas, Texas

CONTENTS

Upper limb amputation is a major disability that interferes with basic activities of daily living and more advanced skills related to employment and leisure activities. A key issue for high-level amputees is how to control movement of their prosthesis. Motorized hooks, hands, wrist units, and elbows are available, but there is no good way for the amputee to "tell" the prosthesis what to do. Target motor reinnervation can produce additional myoelectric control signals for improved powered prosthesis control. This reinnervation allows simultaneous operation of multiple functions in an externally powered prosthesis with physiologically appropriate pathways, and it provides more intuitive control than is possible with conventional myoelectric prostheses.

The present and the future in pediatric prosthetics are bright as a result of ongoing development of new components, materials, and techniques. The focus of clinicians, therapists, and researchers should be to determine the best way of matching components, techniques, and socket designs to the dynamic needs of the child as he or she develops from infant to adult.

In recent years, much attention has been given to the revolution in new materials for prosthetics and the components that they have made possible. The average weight of a delivered prosthesis has decreased, currently available components offer improved function and superior symmetry of gait, and limb interfaces provide superior skin protection and comfort. The focus on the features of these components sometimes has led to neglect of the basic elements of prosthetic design—the fit and the alignment. If the fit and alignment are on the mark, an amputee can function at remarkably high levels with rudimentary components. This article discusses the basics of lower extremity prosthetic practice and addresses challenges for the future.

The availability of advanced materials and techniques means that lower extremity prosthetic users of all ages and amputation levels can achieve a more complete lifestyle recovery. The key component of any lower extremity prosthesis is the socket. The socket is the foundation for the user's comfort, and comfort is the foundation for restoring a person's mobility. Dynamic sockets, "high-tech" liners, and individualized fitting practices are key elements in achieving comfort. Various available suspension systems address the needs of virtually all users. Finally, emerging technologies indicate an even brighter future for all individuals who use a lower extremity prosthesis.

The field of upper extremity prosthetics is a constantly changing arena as researchers and prosthetists strive to bridge the gap between prosthetic reality and upper limb physiology. With the further development of implantable neurologic sensing devices and targeted muscle innervation, the challenge of limited input to control vast outputs promises to become a historical footnote in the future annals of upper limb prosthetics. This article provides readers with basic knowledge of progressive upper limb prosthetics.

The authors compared off-the-shelf (OTS) spinal supports with the custom-molded thoracolumbosacral orthosis (TLSO) in five basic areas: biomechanics, fit, compliance, cost, and liability. Although economically priced OTS orthoses can and should be used under certain prescribed conditions to satisfy carefully described treatment objectives, they cannot control motion as well as custom-molded TLSOs. Patients should not pay for expensive products that cannot help to ensure the best possible clinical outcome. The custom-molded TLSO provides superior fit and support compared to its OTS relative and induces better compliance among its wearers because of its simplicity. It is also the most cost-effective option.

FORTHCOMING ISSUES

RECENT ISSUES

VISIT OUR WEB SITE

The Clinics are now available online!
Access your subscription at www.theclinics.com

PHYSICAL MEDICINE
AND REHABILITATION
CLINICS OF
NORTH AMERICA

Phys Med Rehabil Clin N Am
17 (2006) xi–xii

Foreword

New Advances in Prosthetics and Orthotics

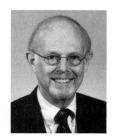

George H. Kraft, MD, MS
Consulting Editor

It has been almost 6 years since the last issue of the *Physical Medicine and Rehabilitation Clinics of North America* devoted to prosthetics and orthotics. In the context of medical care, that is a very long time. There have been many advances in both medicine and engineering since that pre-9/11 era, and this issue reviews them.

Many of the new advances have been in the management of lower limb weakness and amputations. This issue reviews the biomechanical assessment of the lower limb as well as discussing new dynamic lower limb orthoses used to compensate for weakness. Although lower limb amputations are less common than in the past, they still occur, and new developments are discussed. These include new developments in postoperative management, new socket designs and suspensions, new prostheses, and microprocessors for knee units. One of the newest concepts discussed is the use of the Lokomat robotic gait orthosis for gait retraining.

The most striking of the new developments in upper limb prosthetics is the work done on myoelectric designs with myoelectric implants as a means of control. These are discussed in detail by a physician and prosthetist familiar with these topics. Other important topics are also covered. These include scoliosis treatment using spinal orthoses, orthotic management of the limb suffering from neuropathic pain, and the use of prosthetics in pediatric amputations.

1047-9651/06/$ - see front matter © 2006 Elsevier Inc. All rights reserved.

doi:10.1016/j.pmr.2005.12.014

pmr.theclinics.com

The Guest Editor, Dr. Mark Bussell, is both a physician and prosthetist and is uniquely qualified to organize this issue. Readers will recall the excellent August 2000 issue also edited by Dr. Bussell. For this issue, he has recruited a group of experienced writers, including physicians, orthotists, and prosthetists.

I was very pleased when Dr. Bussell accepted my invitation to edit another issue of the *Physical Medicine and Rehabilitation Clinics of North America*. However, it did take some twisting of his arm (perhaps a not inappropriate pun for an issue on prosthetics and orthotics). The readers, however, will be indebted to him for this excellent update, and will be glad I did.

George H. Kraft, MD, MS
Department of Rehabilitation Medicine
University of Washington School of Medicine
1959 NE Pacific Street, Box 356490
Seattle, WA 98195-6490, USA

E-mail address: ghkraft@u.washington.edu

ELSEVIER
SAUNDERS

Phys Med Rehabil Clin N Am
17 (2006) xiii

PHYSICAL MEDICINE
AND REHABILITATION
CLINICS OF
NORTH AMERICA

Preface

New Advances in Prosthetics and Orthotics

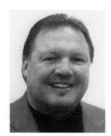

Mark H. Bussell, MD, CPO
Guest Editor

I first met Dr. Kraft in 1979 when I was studying prosthetics and orthotics at the University of Washington. After receiving a Bachelor of Science in Prosthetics and Orthotics, I finished medical school at the University of Illinois at Chicago in 1986. I finished my residency in Physical Medicine and Rehabilitation at Northwestern University's Rehabilitation Institute of Chicago in 1991. I have remained active in the field of prosthetics and orthotics throughout my career.

I was honored when Dr. Kraft asked me to edit another issue of the *Physical Medicine and Rehabilitation Clinics of North America* on prosthetics and orthotics. There have been a plethora of new advances in the field since our last issue in August 2000. I have had the good fortune of meeting and working with many of the country's top experts in the field of prosthetics and orthotics, many of whom have contributed to this issue.

Mark H. Bussell, MD, CPO
7800 Oakmont Boulevard
Fort Worth, TX 76132, USA

E-mail address: docbusman@scglobal.net

1047-9651/06/$ - see front matter © 2006 Elsevier Inc. All rights reserved.
doi:10.1016/j.pmr.2005.11.004

ELSEVIER
SAUNDERS

Phys Med Rehabil Clin N Am
17 (2006) 1–13

PHYSICAL MEDICINE
AND REHABILITATION
CLINICS OF
NORTH AMERICA

Targeted Reinnervation for Improved Prosthetic Function

Todd Kuiken, MD, PhD[a,b,*]

[a]Neural Engineering Center for Artificial Limbs, Rehabilitation Institute of Chicago,
Room 1124, 345 East Superior Street, Chicago, IL 60611, USA
[b]Departments of Physical Medicine Rehabilitation and Biomedical Engineering,
Northwestern University, Chicago, IL 60611, USA

Upper limb amputation is a major disability. It interferes with basic activities of daily living, including dressing, feeding, and personal hygiene, and more advanced skills related to employment and leisure activities. A key issue for high-level amputees is how to control movement of their prosthesis. Motorized hooks, hands, wrist units, and elbows are available, but there is no good way for the amputee to "tell" the prosthesis what to do. Generally, an amputee is able to pull on a single cable with a shoulder harness by protracting the shoulders. This cable can be used to operate one component at a time. When the amputee has positioned one component, he or she activates a switch that locks that component in place, then operates the next component. Alternatively, electromyograms (EMGs) from remaining muscles can be used to control motorized components. Only one component at a time can be operated, however, because of a lack of independent control signals. Sequential control is required to operate a hook or hand, wrist unit, and elbow. At best, body power and external power can be combined for a "hybrid" approach in a transhumeral prosthesis. Current control systems are slow and cumbersome. In short, the treatment options currently available for high-level amputees are severely inadequate.

Although the limb is lost with an amputation, the control signals to the limb remain in the residual peripheral nerves of the amputated limb. An

This article was supported by a Biomedical Engineering Research Grant from the Whitaker Foundation, the National Institute of Child and Human Development (Grants No. 1K08HD01224-01A1, No. 1R01HD043137-01) and the National Institute of Disability and Rehabilitation Research (Grant No. H133G990074-00).

* Neural Engineering Center for Artificial Limbs, Rehabilitation Institute of Chicago, Room 1124, 345 East Superior Street, Chicago, IL 60611, USA.
E-mail address: tkuiken@rehabchicago.org

1047-9651/06/$ - see front matter © 2006 Elsevier Inc. All rights reserved.
doi:10.1016/j.pmr.2005.10.001

appealing concept is to use "neuroelectric control," in which electrodes are connected directly to the residual nerves of the amputee, and the neuroelectric signal is used to control the artificial limb [1–4]. This concept offers the hope of recording from many motor axons to gain additional control information that is related directly to the desired movement of the artificial arm. Signals from wrist flexion motor axons could be used to control a powered wrist flexor, or motor axons to the thenar muscles could be used to operate a powered thumb. Similarly, the afferent fibers might be stimulated to provide sensory feedback of touch, temperature, and position. Dhillon et al [5] showed the potential for the concept of neuroelectric prosthetic control with electrodes temporarily implanted into the residual peripheral nerves of amputees. They successfully recorded motor commands that were usable to control a powered prosthetic hand. These investigators also were able to stimulate axons to give sensory feedback. This work is encouraging, but several inherent problems exist [6]. The neuroelectric signal is very small (microvolts), difficult to record long-term, and difficult to separate from the EMG of surrounding muscle (which has similar frequency content) [7]. Motor nerves also atrophy when they are not connected to muscle, which could compound these problems. A further difficulty arises in transmitting the signals out of the body. This transmission requires either long-term percutaneous wires (which tend to become infected) or complex transmitter-receiver systems. Finally, the durability of the implanted hardware is a crucial issue. Prosthetic control systems are required to function for decades, and neuroelectric control systems would require surgery to repair.

The author has been developing another way to tap into the lost peripheral nerve signals—*targeted reinnervation*. With targeted motor reinnervation, it is possible to denervate expendable regions of muscle in or near an amputated limb and transfer residual arm peripheral nerve endings to these muscles. The nerves reinnervate these muscles. The surface EMG signals from the newly reinnervated muscle can be used as additional control signals for an externally powered prosthesis (Fig. 1).

The main advantages of targeted motor reinnervation are that an increased number of myoelectric control signals are made available, and that these signals relate directly to the original function of the limb. The median, ulnar, musculocutaneous, and radial nerves are present and control different functions in the arm. The EMG signals from muscle reinnervated by these nerves can be used to control functions in the artificial arm that they naturally controlled before amputation. Because each of these nerves innervates muscles that control different, distinct limb motions, they theoretically could supply at least five independent control signals. The median nerve–medial biceps graft can be used to control hand/hook closing. The amputee thinks "close hand," this would send a signal down the median nerve causing reinnervated muscle to contract, and the surface EMG signal from this region could be used to make the motorized hand close. If the patient thinks "bend elbow," this command signal would travel down the

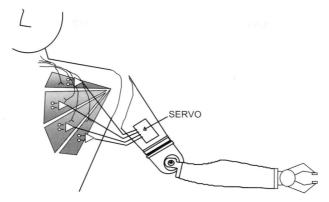

Fig. 1. Conceptual schematic of targeted motor reinnervation.

musculocutaneous nerve, it would cause a different region to contract, and the surface EMG would be used for control of prosthetic elbow flexion. Similarly, the radial nerve can control hand/terminal or elbow extension. The ulnar nerve could control a wrist function, such as wrist rotation or wrist flexion.

With targeted motor reinnervation, the amputee's nerves would control functions in the prosthesis that directly relate to their normal anatomic function. The nerve dominates motor control in the nerve-muscle graft technique so that using the EMG from the nerve transfers as control signals for powered prostheses has a natural feel. Many animal studies have shown that motor control is dominated by the nerve's function in cross-reinnervated muscle, not by the function of the muscle [8,9]. In humans, motor control is strongly dominated by the function of the nerve in cross-reinnervated muscle, but humans are capable of learning to use nerve-muscle grafts in different ways with time and effort [10,11]. When using nerve-muscle grafts for amputees, clinicians would take advantage of the nerve's motor programming so that control of the artificial limb would have a more natural feel than the use of conventional myoelectric prostheses. This motor programming reduces the conscious effort required by the amputee, making the prosthesis easier to use and more functional.

Targeted motor reinnervation need not compromise any other function in the amputee. Only the residual nerves are used, and no functional muscles are denervated with this technique. This technique should not impair shoulder biomechanics further. Shoulder motion still would be available to power or control additional functions in the prosthesis. Using a hybrid approach, additional degrees of freedom could be controlled simultaneously if desired.

Another important advantage of targeted reinnervation is that existing myoelectric technologies could be applied; a new prosthesis would not need to be developed. Powered elbows, wrists, and terminal devices are commercially available. The circuitry is available allowing nine analog inputs (eg, surface EMG signals) and four on/off input signals that provide the control of five motors [12]. The additional control signals would be accessible without the use of implanted nerve cuffs, implanted transmitter-receiver systems, or percutaneous devices that other systems under development may require.

With target sensory reinnervation, it also may be possible to provide physiologically and anatomically appropriate sensory feedback. The concept is to use existing skin in an amputee as a portal to the afferent nerve and provide physiologically appropriate cutaneous feedback. Nerve branches to an area of skin are cut, and the distal end is anastomosed to residual peripheral nerve of the amputee. The afferent fibers now reinnervate this distal nerve segment and then the skin. When the reinnervated skin is touched, it feels like the missing limb is being touched. If a distal cutaneous nerve is anastomosed successfully to the median nerve, when this skin is touched the amputee feels that he or she is being touched somewhere in the palm or first three digits of the hand that is missing. The brain does not know that the skin nerves have been moved, and the brain perceives sensation in whatever territory that the amputated nerve used to innervate. The potential exists to provide light touch, graded pressure, sharp/dull sensation, vibration, and thermal feedback. With appropriate instrumentation, target sensory reinnervation can be used to provide true sensory feedback to amputees. Sensors can be placed in the prosthetic hand so that information is collected about what the prosthesis is touching or how hard it is squeezing (similar to what the Otto Bock Sensor Hand [Otto Bock Health Care, Minneapolis, Minnesota] already does). These data can be used to control actuators that press on or connect to the reinnervated skin of the amputee. An amputee could tell how hard he or she is squeezing with the prosthetic hand or even feel the temperature of his or her coffee.

Requirements for successful implementation of targeted reinnervation

For targeted reinnervation to be successful in amputees, several requirements exist: (1) multiple nerves need to reinnervate separate regions of muscle and skin consistently; (2) independent signals must be recorded from each target area; and (3) a prosthesis must be available that can handle numerous EMG inputs, control multiple motors, and control sensory feedback systems. Previous studies [13,14] found that muscle recovery after nerve transection varies. Such variable recovery could prove problematic for targeted reinnervation. With targeted reinnervation, large nerves containing many times the normal number of motor neurons are transferred onto the muscles, however, "hyperreinnervating" the muscles.

As a first step in the development of this technique, the author tested the hypothesis that hyperreinnervating muscle (transferring an excessive number of motor neurons onto a muscle) would increase the likelihood that any given muscle fiber would be reinnervated and improve muscle recovery

[15]. In this study, rat muscle was hyperreinnervated by grafting additional nerves on to the medial gastrocnemius. Hyperreinnervation significantly improved the recovery of the denervated muscles. The muscle mass and muscle force increased as more motor neurons were grafted on the muscle. In the largest nerve transfers, the experimental muscle recovered to near-normal levels with a relative reinnervation ratio of 94.4% $\pm$ 8.2%, which was significantly greater than the recovery of self-reinnervated muscles ($P < .005$) and was not statistically different from the contralateral unoperated muscles. Based on these results, one can be confident that good muscle recovery would occur with targeted motor reinnervation for amputees.

The efficiency of cutaneous sensory reinnervation is less clear. Similar to targeted muscle reinnervation, hyperreinnervation of skin would be used with targeted sensory reinnervation. A large excess of afferent axons can be transferred to a relatively small area of skin, increasing the likelihood that cutaneous receptors are reinnervated. The cutaneous sensory reinnervation is much more complicated, however, in that there are many types of cutaneous receptors that presumably need to be reinnervated by the correct type of afferent neuron. There are organizational issues because afferent neurons likely do not reinnervate in a pattern reflecting their original cutaneous spatial relationships. More research needs to be done in this area.

Another key issue for the potential success of the targeted reinnervation is myoelectric signal independence. Independent surface EMG signals need to be recorded from each new nerve transfer for control of a prosthesis. The primary measure of myoelectric signal independence is crosstalk between the surface recording sites—the unwanted detection of signals from muscles other than the muscle of interest [16]. For the clinical application of myoelectric prostheses, the electrode is positioned empirically by the prosthetist to the point with the strongest signal and the least crosstalk. Crosstalk can be prevented from interfering with prosthesis operation by setting a threshold; the threshold is set above background noise and the crosstalk from nearby muscles. The amputee must generate an EMG signal greater than the threshold to operate the prosthesis. No published data are available as to what crosstalk levels are acceptable for myoelectric prostheses, but the greater the crosstalk, the higher the threshold must be set, and the harder it is for the amputee to operate the limb. If the threshold is high, it is taxing for the amputee to reach EMG levels above the threshold. This situation is analogous to lifting. If there is too much noise in the first 10 lb of lifting, one considers only the work done from lifting more than 10 lb. It is taxing to lift repeatedly at least 10 lb to do any movement.

Crosstalk depends on many factors, including the geometry of the muscle, the geometry of surrounding tissues such as fat and bone, and the surface recording technique. The author has performed a series of finite element analyses of factors affecting surface EMG signal independence [17–23]. These theoretical estimations present the minimum muscle size from which an independent myoelectric signal can be recorded. Subcutaneous fat was found to be a dominating issue. When subcutaneous fat is minimal (<3 mm), a high degree of signal independence can be expected from recording over a muscle area 2 to 3 cm in diameter. Crosstalk increases between smaller muscles and with thicker subcutaneous fat layers.

Finally, a prosthesis must be available with adequate input channels, sufficient processing power, and the ability to control multiple motors and sensory feedback devices. Until more recently, the Boston Arm (Liberating Technologies, Inc, Holliston, Massachusetts) was the only digital artificial arm with the needed capabilities. It allows nine analog inputs and five digital inputs, it has the needed programming flexibility, and it can control five motors. The Boston Arm has allowed the research team to implement the first generation of targeted reinnervation prostheses.

Initial clinical application

Target reinnervation has been performed successfully in a patient with bilateral shoulder disarticulation [24]. The patient was a 54-year-old white man working as a high-power lineman, who experienced severe electrical burns in May 2002. He initially was fitted with a body-powered prosthesis on the right side and an externally powered prosthesis on the left. A Boston digital arm was operated using four touch pads mounted in the apex of his socket. The patient received extensive training with his prostheses and did well operating the devices by current standards.

The patient had split-thickness skin grafts on both sides of his chest that were hyperesthetic and caused him considerable pain. His local surgeon recommended surgical revision to remove these problematic skin grafts. Because revision surgery was needed, the option of performing targeted muscle reinnervation with transfer of his residual brachial plexus nerves to his pectoralis muscles for improved prosthesis control was discussed. The left limb was chosen because that was the side of his externally powered prosthesis, and the choice was made by the patient and medical team not to change the operation of his right body-powered prosthesis, which worked well for the patient.

This patient was deemed to be a good surgical candidate for multiple reasons. He had good shoulder motion, strong pectoralis muscle contraction, and no sign of brachial plexopathy. The pectoralis muscle, although still under active control, was without function because of the loss of its insertion site on the disarticulated humerus. He had a severe disability and had the potential to gain significant improvement in the operation of his left prosthesis if the targeted muscle reinnervation worked. If the targeted muscle reinnervation failed, his pectoralis muscle would atrophy, but he still would be able to use his prosthesis with the touch pad control. The objective of revising his painful skin graft regions still would be accomplished. Finally, the patient was very intelligent, cooperative, and compliant with his treatment plan.

The goal of surgery was to create four new myoelectric control sites using the four major arm nerves (Fig. 2). During surgery, the split-thickness skin grafts were resected first. Then the four major nerves from the brachial plexus were identified. The native nerve branches to the pectoralis major and minor muscles were cut, and the proximal ends were ligated and sutured up under the clavicle to prevent them from reinnervating the pectoral muscles. The musculocutaneous, median, and radial nerves were transferred on to the clavicular head, the upper sternal head, and the lower sternal head. The pectoralis minor was mobilized out from under the pectoralis major and over to the lateral thoracic wall for two reasons: (1) to serve as a fourth donor muscle segment for the ulnar nerve and (2) to prevent the pectoralis minor EMG from interfering with the myoelectric signals from the other nerve transfers. In each case, the residual plexus nerve was sewn to the native nerve fascicles leading to the muscle and to the muscle itself. Most of the subcutaneous fat was surgically removed over the pectoralis muscles so that the recording electrodes would be as close as possible to the muscle regions of interest with the strongest surface EMG signals possible and the least crosstalk.

The patient recovered from surgery without complication. After approximately 3 weeks, he was able to wear and use his conventional prostheses. As expected, the patient did not have any voluntary active pectoralis contractions after the surgery. After approximately 3 months, the patient noticed his first voluntary "twitches" in his pectoralis muscle when he tried to bend his missing elbow. By 5 months, he could activate four different areas of his pectoralis major muscle. Trying to flex his phantom elbow would cause a strong contraction of the muscle area just beneath the clavicle; this was consistent with musculocutaneous nerve reinnervation. Two separate EMG signals could be detected in the midpectoral region where the

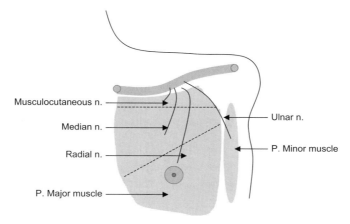

Fig. 2. Diagram of nerve transfers performed in a patient with bilateral shoulder disarticulations.

median nerve–muscle reinnervation was performed. When the patient closed his hand, a good EMG signal could be detected on the lateral pectoral region well below the clavicle. When the patient tried to open his hand, an independent signal could be detected more medially. Because this was an unexpected result, the patient was questioned at length as to what he felt like he was doing to open his hand. He was attempting some thumb abduction movement to generate this signal, but it felt to him like he was naturally trying to open his hand. Extending his elbow and hand caused a palpable contraction of the lower pectoralis muscle, consistent with radial nerve reinnervation. This was a small signal containing a significant electrocardiogram, and the signal was difficult to isolate from the other surface EMG signals. No contraction could ever be appreciated on the lateral chest wall indicating that the ulnar nerve-to-pectoralis minor transfer was unsuccessful.

In addition to the motor reinnervation of the muscle, sensory cross-reinnervation occurred in the skin of the chest wall. When the chest wall was touched in different places, the patient had a sensation of touch to different parts of his hand and arm. The patient had substituted sensation of touch, graded pressure sensation, sharp/dull sensation, and thermal sensation. This sensory cross-reinnervation occurred primarily over the musculocutaneous, median, and ulnar nerve transfers (Fig. 3).

New experimental prostheses were fabricated consisting of a body-powered prosthesis on the right side and the experimental myoelectric prosthesis on the left (Fig. 4). The right-side body-powered prosthesis was unchanged from the initial design with the exception of adding an electronic lock to the shoulder, which was operated by a single touch pad in the apex of the right socket. The left side prosthesis still consisted of a Griefer terminal device (Otto Bock Health Care, Minneapolis, Minnesota), a powered wrist rotator,

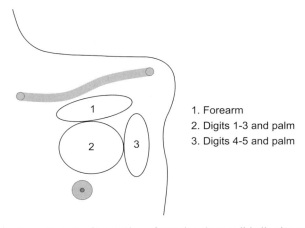

1. Forearm
2. Digits 1-3 and palm
3. Digits 4-5 and palm

Fig. 3. Global pattern sensory reinnervation of anterior chest wall indicating where touching the patient produced sensation in his phantom arm.

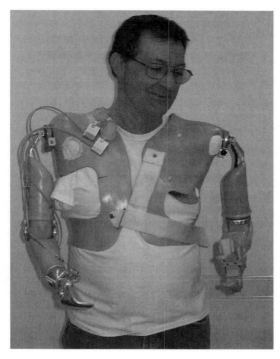

Fig. 4. Experimental prostheses. Left side is an externally powered prosthesis controlled with myoelectric sites created by targeted reinnervation.

a Boston digital arm, and a LTI-Collier Shoulder joint (Liberating Technologies, Inc, Hollistan, Massachusetts). An electronic lock also was added to the left shoulder joint, operated with a single touch pad in the apex of the left socket. The decision was made to use the three most robust EMG signals to control the externally powered prosthesis.

Prosthetic fitting was extremely successful. The patient was able to operate his powered limb with relative ease and markedly improved speed. He also was able to operate his terminal device and his elbow at the same time. He could throw a ball with just the motorized arm. This was the first known demonstration of simultaneous operation of multiple degrees of freedom using only myoelectric control signals.

For objective testing, two tests were performed comparing the function of the touch pad prosthesis with the experimental myoelectric prosthesis. The only standardized and validated test that the team thought was applicable was the box and blocks test [25]. In this test, the subject moves 1-inch square blocks from one box, over a short wall, and into another box. The goal is to see how many blocks the subject can move in 1 minute. The test was modified slightly, allowing the patient 2 minutes to move blocks. The patient showed a 246% increase in speed with his experimental prosthesis. This improvement occurred after using the experimental prosthesis for only 2 months compared with more than 20 months of conventional prosthesis use. A clothespin test was developed that required use of the terminal device, elbow, and wrist rotator unit. In this test, the patient picked up clothespins off of a horizontal bar, rotated the pins, and placed them on a higher vertical bar. The goal was to see how long it took the patient to move three clothespins. On this test, he showed a 26% improvement in speed.

Just as important as the objective testing were the patient's subjective preferences and impressions. The patient reported that he strongly preferred the new myoelectric prosthesis to his previous devices—he felt that there was a "night and day" difference. He found that the myoelectric prosthesis was much easier to use and faster. Perhaps the most telling statement was: "When I use the new prosthesis I just do things—I don't have to think about it." There are numerous tasks that the patient reports he could do better with his new prosthesis and some tasks that he now can do with his new myoelectric prosthesis that he could not do with his previous devices (Table 1). There was one significant problem with the new prosthesis that the patient noted. When he got very sweaty, the prosthesis did not work as well. He needed to take off his prostheses, dry off, and don the devices again, which was a fair amount of work for this patient.

Future research

The case presented here shows the successful use of target reinnervation in a person with shoulder disarticulation amputation. This concept has the potential to benefit individuals with many types of amputation. Currently, the author is conducting a trial of targeted reinnervation in transhumeral amputees. Targeted motor and sensory reinnervation of the median nerve in transradial amputation has the potential to provide thumb control in a multifunction hand and sensory feedback. Targeted reinnervation also may be useful with lower limb amputation. In particular, it could provide

Table 1
Patient's self-report of improved function with nerve-muscle graft controlled prosthesis

Things patient can do *better* with myoelectric prosthesis	*New things* patient can do with myoelectric prosthesis
Take out garbage	Feed himself
Carry groceries	Shave
Pick up yard	Put on socks
Vacuum	Weed in garden
Dust mop	Water the yard
Pick up toys	Open small jar
Put on hat	Use pair of handicap scissors
Put on glasses	Throw a ball
Wash driveway	

information to control a powered ankle with transfemoral amputation and perhaps allow amputees to feel the ground they are walking on better.

The surgical technique for targeted reinnervation might be improved in numerous ways. By splitting the major arm nerves into different parts, it may be possible to create more than one control signal purposefully—as happened by chance with the median nerve in the patient described earlier. Much research needs to be done to understand target sensory reinnervation better and develop useful sensory feedback devices.

Target reinnervation opens the door to many other exciting research possibilities. The ability to control simultaneously more degrees-of-freedom in a prosthesis serves as an impetus to develop new prosthetic components. No motorized shoulder components are currently available for shoulder disarticulation amputees. This is due, at least in part, to inadequate options for controlling such devices. If one has to control sequentially the hand, then the wrist, then the elbow, and then the shoulder, it takes too long, and the cognitive motor planning burden is too high. Target reinnervation would provide better control for such components encouraging their development.

Applying advanced signal processing techniques to the EMG signals from targeted motor reinnervation may lead to further improvements in myoelectric prosthesis control. Many different methods of controlling multiple motions with advanced signal processing techniques have been studied. Although some results have been encouraging, the number of EMG control signals available limits these techniques, especially with high-level amputations. The proposed concept would increase the control information available to these complex decoder algorithms so that they could be applied to high-level amputations with greater success. This increased control information could eliminate the need for surface EMGs over the reinnervated muscles to be completely independent of each other or make it possible to control more than one function in a prosthesis with a single nerve transfer.

Targeted reinnervation also could work synergistically with implantable neural interface systems. The implantable myoelectric sensor (IMES) being developed by Weir et al [26] is a system of small (2×14 mm) implantable telemeter EMG recording devices. They have the potential to enhance significantly the amount and quality of control data with targeted reinnervation subjects. As an implantable electrode, the devices would record for a more localized area, reducing crosstalk issues. A larger number of IMES electrodes could be used than would be practical with surface electrodes. Finally, recording likely would be more stable (ie, less motion artifact and no issues with sweat changing conductance). Targeted reinnervation also could work synergistically with direct nerve recording systems. Having the nerves reinnervate muscle keeps them healthier and more stable. It is likely that neuroelectric control systems may be able to record more and better data for operation of artificial limbs; however, targeted sensory reinnervation is likely to be a better pathway to giving amputees useful sensory feedback. These and other technologies hold great promise on their own and in conjunction with targeted reinnervation.

Summary

Target motor reinnervation can produce additional myoelectric control signals for improved powered prosthesis control. This reinnervation allows simultaneous operation of multiple functions in an externally powered prosthesis with physiologically appropriate pathways, and it provides more intuitive control than is possible with conventional myoelectric prostheses. Target sensory reinnervation has the potential to provide the sensory feedback to the amputee that feels like it is in the missing limb. This concept has great potential for improving the function of people with upper limb amputations, especially for high-level amputations, in which the disability is greatest. It is hoped that future research will develop the technique further and build synergistically with other exciting research areas.

References

[1] Deluca CJ. Control of upper-limb prostheses: a case for neuroelectric control. J Med Eng Tech 1978;2:57–61.

[2] Hoffer JA, Loeb GE. Implantable electrical and mechanical interfaces with nerve and muscle. Ann Biomed Eng 1980;8:351–60.

[3] Edell DE. A peripheral nerve information transducer for amputees: long-term multichannel recordings from rabbit peripheral nerves. IEEE Trans Biomed Eng 1986;33:203–14.

[4] Andrews B. Development of an implanted neural control interface for artificial limbs. Presented at Tenth World Congress of the International Society of Prosthetics and Orthotics. Glasgow, Scotland, July 2001.

[5] Dhillon GS, Lawrence SM, Hutchinson DT, Horch KW. Residual function in peripheral nerve stumps of amputees: implications for neural control of artificial limbs. J Hand Surg Am 2004;29:605–15.

[6] Childress DS. Control of limb prostheses. In: Bowker JH, Michael JW, editors. Atlas of limb prosthetics: surgical, prosthetic, and rehabilitation principles. St. Louis: Mosby Year Book; 1992. p. 175–98.

[7] Upshaw B, Sinkjaer T. Digital signal processing algorithms for the detection of afferent nerve activity recorded from cuff electrodes. IEEE Trans Rehabil Eng 1998;6:172–81.

[8] Sperry RW. The effect of crossing nerves to antagonistic muscle in the hind limb of the rat. J Comp Neurol 1941;75:1–19.

[9] Luff AR, Webb SN. Electromyographic activity in the cross-reinnervated soleus muscle of unrestrained cats. J Physiol 1985;365:13–28.

[10] Nagano A, Tsuyama N, Ochiai N, et al. Direct nerve crossing with the intercostal nerves to treat avulsion injuries of the brachial plexus. J Hand Surg [Am] 1989;14A:980–5.

[11] Clemis JD, Gavron JP. Hypoglossal-facial nerve anastomosis: report on 36 cases with posterior fossa facial paralysis. In: Graham MD, House WF, editors. Disorders of the facial nerve. New York: Raven Press; 1982. p. 499–505.

[12] Williams T.W. New control options for upper limb prostheses. Presented at the Tenth World Congress of the International Society of Prosthetics and Orthotics. Glasgow, Scotland, July 2001.

[13] Frey M, Gruber H, Holle J, Freilinger G. An experimental comparison of the different kinds of muscle reinnervation: nerve suture, nerve implantation, and muscular neurotization. Plast Reconstr Surg 1982;69:656–67.

[14] Gordon T, Stein RB. Time course and extent of recovery in reinnervated motor units of cat triceps surae muscles. J Physiol [E] 1982;323:307–23.

[15] Kuiken TA, Rymer WZ, Childress DS. The hyper-reinnervation of rat skeletal muscle. Brain Res 1995;676:113–23.

[16] Lowery MM, Stoykov NS, Taflove A, Kuiken TA. An analysis of surface EMG signal independence. IEEE Trans Biomed Eng 2003;50(6):789–93.

[17] Stoykov NS, Lowery MM, Kuiken TA. A finite-element analysis of the effect of muscle insulation and shielding on the surface EMG signal. IEEE Trans Biomed Eng 2005;52(1): 117–21.

[18] Lowery MM, Stoykov NS, Dewald JPA, Kuiken TA. Volume conduction in an anatomically-based surface EMG model. IEEE Trans Biomed Eng 2004;51(12):2138–47.

[19] Lowery MM, Stoykov NS, Kuiken TA. Independence of myoelectric control signals examined using a surface EMG model. IEEE Trans Biomed Eng 2003;50:789–93.

[20] Kuiken TA, Lowery MM, Stoykov NS. The effect of subcutaneous fat on myoelectric signal amplitude and cross-talk. Prosthet Orthot Int 2003;27:48–54.

[21] Lowery MM, Stoykov NS, Taflove A, Kuiken TA. A simulation study of surface EMG cross-talk as an estimate of surface EMG cross-talk. J Appl Physiol 2003;94:1324–34.

[22] Lowery MM, Stoykov NS, Taflove A, Kuiken TA. A multi-layer finite element model of the surface EMG signal. IEEE Trans Biomed Eng 2002;49:446–54.

[23] Kuiken TA, Stoykov NS, Popovic M, et al. Finite element modelling of electromagnetic signal propagation in a phantom arm. IEEE Trans Neural Syst Rehabil Eng 2001;9:346–54.

[24] Kuiken TA, Dumanian GA, Lipschutz RD, et al. The use of targeted muscle reinnervation for improved myoelectric prosthesis control in a bilateral shoulder disarticulation amputee. Prosthet Orthot Int 2004;28(3):245–53.

[25] Mathiowetz V, Volland G, Kashman N, Weber K. Adult norms for the box and blocks test of manual dexterity. Am J Occup Ther 1985;39:386–91.

[26] Weir RF, Troyk PR, DeMichele G, Kuiken TA. Implantable myoelectric sensors (IMES) for upper-extremity prosthesis control—preliminary work. Presented at Twenty-fifth Annual Conference of the IEEE EMBS. Cancun, Mexico, 2003.

ELSEVIER
SAUNDERS

Phys Med Rehabil Clin N Am
17 (2006) 15–21

PHYSICAL MEDICINE
AND REHABILITATION
CLINICS OF
NORTH AMERICA

Pediatric Prosthetics: An Update

Donald R. Cummings, CP (LP)

Department of Prosthetics, Texas Scottish Rite Hospital for Children,
2222 Welborn, Dallas, TX 75219

Innovative prosthetic components, materials, and technologic advances continue to expand the options available to pediatric amputees. Successful socket design always has been the first priority for prosthetists regardless of the age of the patient for whom they are fitting a prosthesis. If the socket—the interface between the child with an amputation and the prosthesis—is not fitted comfortably and functionally, it negates the benefits of even the most sophisticated components and materials. In pediatrics, socket design is complicated by the need to address the child's growth and development. Socks, flexible inner sockets, gel or foam liners, and frequent follow-up all are routine methods of dealing with growth changes. Alignment—the establishment of the optimal biomechanical relationship between the prosthetic components and the patient—is probably second in importance, followed by materials, components, and cosmetic appearance. All of these features are interrelated, however. A particular child's comfort might be enhanced through a protective gel liner and a flexible inner socket, which might be bulky enough to detract from the cosmetic appearance of the limb. Socket design and materials also may influence the performance and selection of components such as knees, ankles, and feet.

The design process inevitably involves choice. Although adult amputees make many choices regarding their prosthetic design, for young children, it is usually the parents and the clinical team who choose. A crucial part of the pediatric prosthetist's role is to educate parents and the clinical team about socket design options and how they influence and relate to the rest of the prosthesis and to how soon the device may need to be replaced because of growth and wear and tear. Regardless, children 5 years old and younger generally require a new prosthesis annually, then biannually from age 5 to 12 years, and then once every 3 or 4 years thereafter [1].

E-mail address: Don.Cummings@tsrh.org

1047-9651/06/$ - see front matter © 2006 Elsevier Inc. All rights reserved.

doi:10.1016/j.pmr.2005.10.002

Unique aspects of prosthetic design as they relate to children were described in a 2000 issue of the *Physical Medicine and Rehabilitation Clinics of North America* [2]. These aspects included staging components, designs and alignment based on development, accommodating growth changes, greater frequency of Syme's (ankle disarticulation) and knee disarticulation fittings, adjusting for overgrowth in transdiaphyseal amputations, and common surgical revisions such as correcting angular deformity or revising terminal bone overgrowth. These key considerations have not changed significantly, but newer "adult" prosthetic techniques have influenced how they are managed. Such evolving advances include computer-aided design; multiple above-knee ischial-containment socket versions; and multiple total surface bearing strategies using various silicone, urethane, or thermoplastic gel liners for comfort, limb protection, and suspension. All of these approaches and components have been well described elsewhere [3–7]. There is a bit of a "trickle-down" effect because innovations generally are aimed at the larger adult market first, then gradually are modified to address fittings for children. Most are being adapted or modified gradually for pediatric application, which usually means they are smaller in scale, and their biomechanical principles are applied less aggressively. In general, these design approaches reflect an industry that is maturing in its understanding of the biomechanical needs of each patient; of use of a growing body of related research; and of sound use of materials, components and techniques to meet patients' needs.

Components and materials

Prosthetic components—items such as feet, knees, pylons, adaptors, liners, socks, hands, wrists, and electrodes—often are prefabricated products that the prosthetist builds into the prosthesis. Today (disproportionately more for adults than children), there is a dazzling array of such products available from numerous manufacturers and suppliers. Essentially, prosthetic components are merely parts—the "nuts and bolts" of the device. To benefit a patient, components should be selected appropriately, matched with a properly made and fitted socket, aligned according to appropriate biomechanical methods, and assembled and maintained according to the manufacturer's specifications. The patient or the caregivers should be educated about the entire device, including how the components function, precautions, and any special care and maintenance that may be required.

It is well understood that children with limb deficiencies, particularly children with multiple limb involvement, have problems that differ from adult amputees [8]. In addition to their limb deficiencies, from birth until skeletal maturity, children experience normal, often rapid changes in their neurologic development, muscle strength, skeletal alignment, height, center of gravity, and gait [9,10]. Simply downsizing adult components for pediatric use may miss the mark. This situation frequently presents a problem for researchers, manufacturers, and entrepreneurs in the business of developing prosthetic components. The pediatric "market" is much smaller than the adult one, yet costs for research and development of new components are relatively the same. It is often not economically feasible for manufacturers to develop, produce, and stock multiple sizes and specialized variations of prosthetic components that have a small turnover. Practitioners who make prostheses for children frequently have far fewer choices of feet, knees, socks, liners, and sleeves to choose from than do practitioners who work primarily with adults. Many components simply are not available in a pediatric version. A pediatric prosthetist commonly has to modify an existing adult component significantly or custom make components to meet the unique needs of a pediatric client. This situation is gradually improving, however.

In recent years, consumer demand, competition, and interest on the part of manufacturers to address the pediatric "niche" market have led several companies to develop complete lines of pediatric components "from the ground up." Today, most prosthetic supplier catalogs include a separate section for pediatric prosthetic components for upper and lower limbs. One rationale for this trend is that if a child develops a preference for a certain component and its appearance and feel, the child may continue to prefer that component (or similar versions) on into adulthood. This approach is appealing to prosthetists as long as they can be assured components are appropriately designed and tested for children's weights, sizes, and activities throughout their growing years.

Examples of some specific product advances in pediatrics include more energy storing and release feet and feet with energy storing and release capabilities and multiaxial ankle function. At the time this article is being written, at least six manufacturers supply prosthetic feet in these categories, in sizes as small as 14 cm in length. Several manufacturers include adaptors or disks in graduated sizes so that prosthetists can lengthen the prosthesis easily as the child grows. Most include foot shells with cosmetic toes, two or more skin tones, multiple attachment hardware options, and the ability to select ankle and foot "stiffness." What specific functional benefits these feet provide for adults and children is still the subject of debate and much ongoing research [11–13].

In the United States, modular prosthetic knees for children, particularly several popular polycentric versions, largely have reduced use of traditional single-axis, exoskeletal designs. Depending on the manufacturer, such knees possess the advantages of the increased stability associated with multiaxial knees, adjustable friction, extension-assist springs, stance phase resistance to buckling, and modularity and are often small enough to be used with children 2 years old. Prosthetic knees with a rubberized knee cap seem to be preferred because they facilitate kneeling; save wear and tear on clothing and floors; and can be finished with durable, "open knee" or "discontinuous" covers frequently used with children and adolescents.

Microprocessor-controlled knees have captured headlines and the imagination of the public. The efficacy of microprocessor-controlled knees for the younger population has not been documented because none are designed for small children. For adolescents and young adults, these knees may provide many of the same advantages that adult users report, including greater ease of walking at various speeds, improved stability and confidence descending slopes, and more natural knee responsiveness [14]. Most of these components still are not recommended for highly active patients; yet by definition, because they tend to run, compete athletically, and participate in water-related activities, most adolescent amputees fall into the highest functional ambulation category. This is a case in which time, movement science studies, and eventual filtering down of the technology into pediatrics will determine how these systems best benefit the pediatric population.

Gel liners are an accepted component in general prosthetic practice as a means of protecting the limb and suspending the prosthesis. These liners come in multiple sizes, thicknesses, shapes, and materials from numerous manufacturers and have been well described. In pediatrics, liners sometimes offer the added advantage of allowing the prosthetist to adjust for a child's growth by switching to a thinner liner or reducing the thickness of socks worn over the liner. Many prosthetists use them for upper and lower limb prostheses. The use of silicon, urethane, or mineral oil–based thermoplastic gel liners in pediatrics continues to increase as various manufacturers offer smaller sizes and appropriate pins, shuttle locks, lanyards, suction valves, and other suspension adaptors. One liner, now available in sizes small enough for many children, has a unique circumferential membrane on the outside, lower portion of the liner. When used in combination with a socket and distal air-expulsion valve, the membrane provides excellent suction. The author has found this system to work well as a means of suspending transtibial and knee-disarticulation prostheses for some children.

Most prosthetists have the capability to manufacture customized silicon gel liners, but the process can be time-consuming,and it is difficult to manufacture successfully replacement liners that are exactly the same thickness. Several companies offer a customized service that enables the prosthetist to specify, either on a cast or a digitized image, the location and thickness of gel. In some cases, regions of gel with a different durometer can be combined into one liner. When a mold is fabricated or stored in memory, the liner can be duplicated or modified as needed. This process is slightly more costly, but enables some challenging limbs, such as limbs with burns, scars, angular deformities, or unusually sharp bony prominences, to be fitted more successfully.

Many of the components and product developments just described have a downside. They are better matched to growing children and their size, weight, and activity level than in prior years and provide more options for pediatric clients, but most come with time-based warranties and specific patient weight and activity parameters, torque settings, and maintenance schedules. Such factors can influence how frequently components or the entire prosthesis must be replaced.

Newer and better materials have had a positive influence on pediatric prosthetic fitting. Examples include silicones and urethanes, which can be used as interfaces and protective pads. Thermoplastics, particularly those that can be used to fabricate flexible inner sockets, continue to provide benefits to children. Sockets fabricated from such materials may provide sufficient flexibility to make it easier for a child to don and doff a prosthesis over a bulbous distal end, as with an ankle or knee disarticulation. The prosthetist often can heat and stretch a flexible socket easily to adjust for growth or heat and shrink it as a limb loses volume through reduction of swelling or atrophy. Lighter and stronger materials with unique properties continue to be developed for use in other industries and adapted for prosthetic use.

Upper limb prosthetics

To cover the broad array of component choices and changing technology in upper limb prosthetics is beyond the scope of this article. General advancements in upper limb prosthetics, particularly powered systems, also are well described in the article by Lake elsewhere in this issue.

From a philosophical perspective, an observable change in recent years has been gradual acceptance among pediatric prosthetic fitting centers of a broader age range during which fitting an upper limb prosthesis is appropriate. The age considered "ideal" is usually a reflection of the philosophy of a center that fits a lot of upper limb prostheses for children. The clinic's approach may be influenced by the degree of access their patients have to adequate funding, occupational therapy, and prosthetic adjustments and maintenance. The fact that some centers are fitting infants 4 or 5 months old with either a passive or a myoelectric arm is no longer as controversial a practice as it once was. In general, however, the tenets of the past 25 years or so are still followed: If the family has opted for prosthetic fitting, the child is fitted with a passive device when he or she begins to gain sitting balance (usually 4–6 months old). By age 2 years, if the child is still routinely wearing the device, training the child with an activated terminal device, such as a single-site myoelectric hand or a body-powered device, is begun [15].

Externally powered prostheses are not the only focus of development. Body-powered hooks and their variants still are considered among the most functional of terminal devices. Traditionally, hooks have been valued for their ability to grasp small and large objects with precision; the fact that they do not block the user's view of objects, as do prosthetic hands; their low cost; high durability; and appropriateness for labor and leisure activities [16]. Devices that are more "hooklike" in function have been designed to include cosmetic features that help them appear more like a hand. In effect, the thumb and first two fingers grasp via a harness and cable system, and the fourth and fifth "fingers" are sculpted into the rubber or urethane to make them appear to have been flexed into the "palm" of the device.

Access to information

As a result of access to the Internet, consumer groups, and disability-specific publications and websites, today's prosthetic patient or family members often have done considerable research regarding the patient's condition before the first appointment with a prosthetist. This is a positive trend because in general an educated patient or family members make better choices regarding prosthetic options, components, surgical approaches, and therapy.

Gaps in progress

Today's pediatric prosthetists and the patients they serve still could benefit from improved methods of cosmetic finishing with a much higher degree of durability. Fluid-controlled knees that are smaller and lighter than current versions likely would benefit patients age 4 years and older who are actively running. Feet and knees truly designed for children younger than age 4 would be an improvement if they were smaller and lighter and took up less space. Many prosthetic components, particularly knees, feet, and shuttle lock systems, could be improved if they were made waterproof. Children and parents frequently complain that many parts of the prosthesis are easily damaged by water, yet children love to play in the water. Feet and attachment hardware with a shorter "build height" to fit within the relatively small space available for young patients with ankle disarticulations are needed. Lawn mower injuries are among the most common causes for partial foot amputations in children, yet levels such as the Chopart amputation continue to be technically difficult to fit, and few components exist. In the upper limb, partial hand and finger amputations are among the most common levels, but few prostheses and specialized components and techniques exist for these levels, particularly for children. For higher levels, hands with more degrees of freedom and smaller, lighter batteries and motors are needed. Prosthetic hand function could be improved through the development of gloves that are far more durable and have the ability to stretch in a natural way, enhancing efficiency of motors. Sensory feedback for prosthetic hands is still a major, yet elusive priority for children and researchers. Ideally, motor control and sensory feedback through either the central nervous system or peripheral nerve connections will become available.

Summary

The present and the future in pediatric prosthetics are bright as a result of ongoing development of new components, materials, and techniques. The focus of clinicians, therapists, and researchers should be to determine the best way of matching components, techniques, and socket designs to the dynamic needs of the child as he or she develops from infant to adult.

Resources

1. Amputee Coalition of America (ACA). Available at: www.amputee-coalition.org (1-888-267-5669).
2. Association of Children's Prosthetic Orthotic Clinics (ACPOC). Available at: www.acpoc.org (1-847-384-4226).
3. Herring J, Birch J, editors. The child with a limb deficiency. Rosemont (IL): American Academy of Orthopaedic Surgeons; 1997.
4. Muzumdar A, Herring J, editors. Powered upper limb prostheses, control implementation and clinical application. Berlin: Springer-Verlag; 2004.
5. Orthotics and prosthetics.com. Available at: http://www.oandp.com/.

References

[1] Lambert C. Amputation surgery in the child. Orthop Clin North Am 1972;3:473–82.
[2] Cummings D. Pediatric prosthetics: current trends and future possibilities. Phys Med Rehabil Clin N Am 2000;11:653–79.
[3] Brncick M. Computer automated design and computer automated manufacture. Phys Med Rehabil Clin N Am 2000;11:701–4.
[4] Edwards M. Below knee socket designs and suspension systems. Phys Med Rehabil Clin N Am 2000;11:585–93.
[5] Herring J, editor. Limb deficiencies. In: Tachdjian's pediatric orthopedics. 3rd edition. Philadelphia: Saunders; 2002. p. 1745–810.
[6] Kapp S. Transfemoral socket designs and suspension options. Phys Med Rehabil Clin N Am 2000;11:569–83.
[7] Michael J. Prosthetic suspensions and components. In: Smith D, Michael J, Bowker J, editors. Atlas of amputations and limb deficiencies, surgical, prosthetic and rehabilitation principles. 3rd edition. Rosemont (IL): American Academy of Orthopaedic Surgeons; 2004. p. 409–27.
[8] Watts H. Multiple limb deficiencies. In: Smith D, Michael J, Bowker J, editors. Atlas of amputations and limb deficiencies, surgical, prosthetic and rehabilitation principles. 3rd edition. Rosemont (IL): American Academy of Orthopaedic Surgeons; 2004. p. 923–9.
[9] Sutherland D, Olshen R, Biden E, Wyatt M. The development of mature walking. London: Mac Keith Press; 1988.
[10] Sutherland D. Review paper: the development of mature gait. Gait Posture 1997;6:163–70.
[11] Hafner B, Sanders J, Czerniecki J, et al. Energy storage and return prostheses: does patient perception correlate with biomechanical analysis? Clin Biomech 2002;17:325–44.
[12] Menard M, McBride ME, Sanderson D, Murray DD. Comparative biomechanical analysis of energy-storing prosthetic feet. Arch Phys Med Rehabil 1992;73:451–8.
[13] Perry J. Amputee gait. In: Smith D, Michael J, Bowker J, editors. Atlas of amputations and limb deficiencies, surgical, prosthetic and rehabilitation principles. 3rd edition. Rosemont (IL): American Academy of Orthopaedic Surgeons; 2004. p. 367–84.
[14] Friel K. Componentry for lower extremity prostheses. J Am Acad Orthop Surg 2005;13:326–35.
[15] Patton J. Occupational therapy. In: Smith D, Michael J, Bowker J, editors. Atlas of amputations and limb deficiencies, surgical, prosthetic and rehabilitation principles. 3rd edition. Rosemont (IL): American Academy of Orthopaedic Surgeons; 2004. p. 813–29.
[16] Atkins DJ, Donovan WH, Heard D, et al. Current trends in fitting the child with an upper limb deficiency and implications for further prosthetic research [abstract]. Orthop Trans 1995;123:19.

ELSEVIER
SAUNDERS

Phys Med Rehabil Clin N Am
17 (2006) 23–30

PHYSICAL MEDICINE
AND REHABILITATION
CLINICS OF
NORTH AMERICA

Changes in Lower Extremity Prosthetic Practice

Ted A. Trower, CPO

A-S-C Orthotics & Prosthetics, 1407 East Michigan Avenue, Jackson, MI 49202, USA

"If the socket doesn't fit, and isn't aligned right, the amp will sit."
—Honorable John J. Farley III, US Court of Appeals (Ret.)

In recent years, much attention has been given to the revolution in new materials for prosthetics and the components that they have made possible. The average weight of a delivered prosthesis has decreased on the order of 50% to 75% since the author began practice in 1981. Currently available components offer improved function and superior symmetry of gait. Limb interfaces provide superior skin protection and comfort. The focus on the features of these components sometimes has led, however, to neglect of the basic elements of prosthetic design—the fit and the alignment. Any experienced prosthetist has seen the evidence that if the fit and alignment are on the mark, an amputee can function at remarkably high levels with rudimentary components, even with obsolete components such as the SACH (Solid Ankle Cushion Heel) foot.

What is lacking is a superior understanding of what it is that makes a socket "fit." The fundamental principles of total contact, uniform pressure distribution, elimination of shear stress and focal pressures, and restoration of correct limb length have been known for a long time. The past decades have seen many studies of socket pressures, vascular flow, muscle activity, tissue density, measurement techniques, fabrication materials, and methods. None of these studies has shown a way to consistently produce a comfortable, stable fit and alignment without the need for trial-and-error fittings.

There have been improvements in the quality of the fit delivered to amputees. Although the use of test sockets was relatively uncommon in the early 1980s, the practice of using multiple transparent test sockets is widely accepted today. This process of trial and error yields a superior result, but does not reflect a superior understanding of *why* a socket fits well. Socket

E-mail address: ted@amputee.com

1047-9651/06/$ - see front matter © 2006 Elsevier Inc. All rights reserved.
doi:10.1016/j.pmr.2005.10.003

pmr.theclinics.com

design has continued to evolve, and some truly creative new designs have been introduced. These designs do not reflect a superior understanding, however, of what synergy of support, compression, alignment, and flexibility would offer the maximum in comfort and function. Today's sockets are produced in the same empirical manner as their predecessors. Previous experience is the still best tool available in producing a comfortable fitting socket because clinicians do not have the knowledge to create one based on scientific procedures.

The use of multiple test fittings allows more opportunities for, and range of, adjustment in the process of static and dynamic alignment. The improved quality of fit provides a more stable interface between the residual limb and the prosthetic socket. This stable interface translates to improved control of the prosthesis and reduced torques applied on the residual limb. This improvement is fortunate because alignment issues have received little attention in the literature in recent years. There has been a trend to neglect alignment needs in service to component selection. The increase in the use of pin-lock suspensions has often been the villain in this case. Many manufacturers of pin-lock mechanisms produced them with a modular pyramid connector attached to their distal surface. This type of mechanism is appealing if efficiency of production is a concern. Numerous prosthetists have allowed this hardware design to dictate the alignment of the prostheses they fitted. When using a lock with the pyramid connector at the distal end of the locking mechanism, the prosthetist is forced to position the proximal end of the prosthetic pylon directly under the distal end of the socket. This positioning limits the placement of the prosthetic foot to the narrow range of positions allowed by the limits of the adjustment range of the endoskeletal system in use. In some cases, this is an entirely satisfactory result, but more often it causes the foot to be positioned too far posteriorly and or too far laterally for optimal function and stability. This is an entirely unnecessary problem because many pin-lock mechanisms are available without the pyramid attached, and fabrication of a socket in a proper alignment is readily accomplished with any of them. The parameters that determine proper alignment are independent of the components used in the construction of the prosthesis with the possible exceptions of some prosthetic knee units and the feet designed with excessively short keels or hard heels.

Prosthetic socket design has seen the introduction of many new ideas and techniques. New fabrication materials and measurement techniques lead the list of widely accepted improvements over previous methods. Measurement and molding techniques have seen numerous changes. Although traditional plaster casting still is the most common method for obtaining a mold of the residual limb, other options are growing rapidly in popularity. In a minor variation of technique, some prosthetists are using fiberglass casting materials to obtain their molds. These materials set more rapidly and capture less detail, but are effective and timesaving. More dramatic are the techniques used to capture a digital model for use in computer-assisted design/

computer-assisted manufacturing (CAD/CAM) socket production systems. Although mechanical digitizers that trace the interior of a traditional plaster cast are still most common, a variety of techniques are being used to input the digital mold of an amputee's limb. Electromagnetic wands that trace the surface of the limb and optical systems that use lasers or high-contrast garments to accentuate contours for video capture show great promise and offer the hope of a prosthetic facility completely free of plaster mess and expense. The superiority of any one system for capture of digital models has yet to be proved, and it may prove to be that each one will find its place in the practice of prosthetics. Digital socket models have led to the availability of "digital test sockets." These are conventional transparent test sockets fabricated in a CAD/CAM system from measurements only, without the benefit of a three-dimensional model of the actual amputee. They are reported to be generally successful when used for fitting the transfemoral residual limb. One point about this technique is that it harkens back to the days of the wood socket when measurements were the only data available for use in fabrication of a socket.

Along with measurement techniques, socket design has undergone changes. The traditional patellar tendon bearing (PTB) socket design is rarely seen today. Its descendent has softened contours and a much less pronounced loading of the patellar ligament. With the widespread use of gel liners in transtibial sockets, the PTB has evolved in the direction of the total surface bearing (TSB) design. True TSB fitting requires uniform loading of all tissues, and in the author's experience, it is rarely successful because of the instability of residual limb volume on a day-to-day basis. More practical, and successful, fittings incorporate elements of the PTB and the TSB designs. Total contact within the socket is essential, and all tissues must carry some loading. Selectively applied increased loading of load-tolerant tissues and reduced loading of sensitive tissues are necessary to prevent injury when limb volume decreases, and the residual limb drops more deeply onto the socket than is desired. The changes in limb contour that occur with fluid volume fluctuation are not distributed uniformly, but rather are concentrated in the areas of the soft tissue masses. Because many skeletal structures in the transtibial residual limb are close to the skin surface, they are exposed to carrying an increased weight-bearing load when the load borne on the soft tissue areas is reduced.

Although the changes to transtibial socket design have been incremental, the changes in transfemoral socket design have been significant and dramatic. The period after the introduction of ischial containment sockets has been one of anarchy with regard to socket design. Several different transfemoral socket designs have been promoted and taught, but none were consistently successful without each prosthetist adapting the technique to his or her own methods, often to the point that the elements of the original design were difficult to identify. The socket styles used for transfemoral amputee fittings have been so widely varied and individual that it frequently has been possible to identify which prosthetist created the socket just by examining the socket contours and trimlines.

The most recently introduced design promises to bring order to the universe of transfemoral fittings. The Marlo Anatomical Socket (MAS), also commonly referred to as a Marlo socket, was developed by Marlo Ortiz Vazquez of Jalisco, Mexico. The principles and the procedures for the creation of the MAS have been clarified and outlined by John Michael of CPO Services, Inc (Portage, Indiana). This design is a remarkable step forward in prosthetic fitting technology. The MAS socket provides ischial containment and mediolateral stability superior to previous designs, while providing reduced trimlines, greater range of motion, increased comfort, and the potential for superb cosmetic finishing. The design has proved to be readily teachable. The MAS is one of the few socket designs for which the training course has proved effective in transmitting the necessary information for successful implementation. This is not a contradiction of the earlier statement that why a socket fits or does not fit is unknown. The MAS design still requires test fittings, and fittings do improve with the experience of the prosthetist. The MAS seminar comes closer to teaching a successful technique than any other socket course in the author's experience.

The most striking feature of the MAS socket is the ischial-ramal containment (IRC) extension. This structure is not designed to provide a weight-bearing surface for the ischial tuberosity as is done in most ischial containment sockets. The IRC extension is intended to be positioned immediately medial to, and parallel with, the pubic ramus and the ischial tuberosity. It provides a structural limit to lateral displacement of the proximal socket. On first examination, it appears to extend unreasonably high into the perineum, but this is not the case. The IRC extension appears to extend so high because the surrounding structures of the socket have been lowered to provide increased comfort and range of motion. The reduction in the height of the posterior brim of the socket also improves the cosmesis in that area by reducing the unnatural elevation of the tissues of the buttock. By placing a traditional ischial containment socket alongside a MAS socket fitted to the same amputee, one can see that the IRC extension is elevated to almost exactly the same height as the ischial region of the ischial containment socket. Because the IRC extension of the MAS is not weight bearing, and because its contours are more narrow and more rounded, it is much more comfortable to wear than a traditional ischial containment/ischial weight-bearing design.

First popularized as a part of the ISNY (Icelandic-Scandinavian-New York) design, flexible thermoplastic sockets with rigid external frames are commonly used today, especially in transfemoral fittings. A wide range of plastic materials is available allowing the prosthetist to select the desired degree of stiffness or flexibility according to need or preference. New, more flexible plastics allow muscles to expand in circumference as they contract in length to a much greater degree than did the original polyethylene. Other plastics provide structural support and do not require any external frame at all.

Carbon fiber reinforcement was previously an expensive curiosity. Applying the material was labor intensive and complex. The availability of carbon fiber in braided tubes has simplified its use greatly, and the costs have decreased with increased application. Today, it is common to see sockets fabricated of carbon fiber alone. Many different resins and resin blends based on epoxies or acrylics or both are now available. Each has differing properties, but all offer strength and impact resistance far superior to the old, and no longer available, 4110 polyester resin.

CAD/CAM systems, first introduced at the ISPO World Congress in 1983, have increased in number and sophistication over time. Today, many prosthetic facilities use CAD/CAM for all but their most unusual fittings, such as some congenital anomalies with irregular shaped limbs. Although some clinicians have touted CAD/CAM as a superior way to fit a prosthesis, there is no evidence that this is true in the area of quality of fit obtained. There are some production efficiencies to be had using CAD/CAM in high-volume environments. Sometimes criticized as a way to make mistakes with greater precision, the "high tech" of CAD/CAM has not yet helped clinicians to answer the question of why a socket fits well. Even in the highly technical world of digital limb modeling, the technique remains empirical. We know how to make a socket fit, we know how to assess when a socket fits, but we do not know why it fits or why it fails.

The introduction of roll-on gel liners has had a large impact on lower extremity prosthetic practice at all levels with the exceptions of partial feet and hip disarticulation/hemipelvectomy. At the transtibial and the transfemoral levels, the use of gel liners for comfort or suspension or both has become normal practice. Gel liners come in three primary materials—silicone, thermoplastic polymer, and urethane. They can be custom fabricated, but most in use are prefabricated designs. The liners of thermoplastic polymer can be customized to some degree by heating while stretched over a plaster or plastic model; this results in thinning of the liner over prominent structures, precisely the locations that would benefit most from a heavier layer of gel cushioning. Silicone and urethane liners seem to be more durable than liners made of thermoplastic gels. Urethane liners tend to discolor over time and can become sticky to touch as they deteriorate. Silicone is more expensive, but many clinicians believe that the extra expense is worthwhile. All roll-on gel liners require excellent hygiene for the prevention of discoloration of the liner, odors, and bacterial or fungal skin infections. The primary contraindication to their use is poor personal hygiene and noncompliance with liner hygiene requirements. When applied to a conscientious and hygienic individual, roll-on gel liners offer improved soft tissue protection and comfort. They also offer the option for use as a suspension system and are extremely effective for this application. More recently, Ossur (Aliso Viejo, California) has introduced a roll-on liner that uses a circumferential gasket to provide a suction suspension reminiscent of the hypobaric sock. This liner has proved to be successful in transfemoral fittings. The effectiveness in transtibial fittings remains to be seen. The advantages of this system include ease of donning and the ability to adjust fit using socks, while retaining the effectiveness of a suction suspension. Roll-on liners with locking pins or lanyard straps positioned distally have altered prosthetic fitting patterns dramatically. Waist belts and cuff straps now are used far less commonly. Conventional suction socket transfemoral fittings also are fading rapidly out of usage. Locking/lanyard suspensions offer greatly increased ease of donning and the ability to adjust socket fit for volume changes through the use of limb socks.

One area of prosthetic hardware that has seen dramatic and rapid changes is that of knee control units, specifically, the introduction of microprocessor controlled knee units. These are addressed in the article by Berry elsewhere in this issue and are not described here except to acknowledge that with careful selection of candidates for fitting, they seem to offer superior function for normal activities of daily living, but they do not seem to be well suited to athletic individuals or endeavors. It is reasonable to believe that the pattern of acceptance and improvement that has been witnessed since the 1980s in the realm of dynamic response feet is likely to repeated in the next 2 decades by the microprocessor controlled knee units. Twenty years after their introduction, dynamic response feet have taken their place in the mainstream of prosthetic practice. They now come in a large variety of forms from high-performance feet for athletic competition to low-profile designs that incorporate multiaxial movement to designs that allow the dispersal of vertical impact and torsion forces.

Component hardware and socket design are not the only elements of prosthetics that have been changing. Attitudes toward prostheses are changing among consumers and the public. Amputees today decry the use of the term *patient,* arguing that they are not ill and do not require treatment. Educated consumers think of themselves as clients to their prosthetists, and amputees are much more educated than they have ever been before. The Internet has created an opportunity for individuals who previously were isolated by geography to communicate daily at little cost. They can compare notes on issues with fellow amputees, whereas previously they would have been completely dependent on the professionals providing their care. Organizations such as the Amputee Coalition of America have made tremendous amounts of information available on the World Wide Web. Manufacturers of prosthetic components have recognized the value of educating their end consumers and now mount major marketing efforts targeting amputees directly instead of directing their attention only to the professional caregiver. Society as a whole is more accepting of public visibility of disabled individuals, and the disabled community is striving for even greater acceptance. In the prosthetic arena, this is seen in the movement away from efforts to conceal a prosthesis behind cosmetic shaping or coloration. The *New York*

Times has taken note of this trend [1]. Use of colorful decorative laminations is becoming much more common and is no longer limited to young or flamboyant individuals.

Not all of the societal changes in the field of prosthetics have been improvements. Managed care continues to protect insurance company profits by creating barriers to access to care. Short-term thinking by third-party payers frequently leads to nonsensical decisions, such as refusing minor repairs or necessary accessories. Medicare functional level guidelines deny dynamic response foot components to the challenged individuals who would most benefit from their efficiency and lightweight construction. Manufacturers of prosthetic components are undergoing a period of consolidation and acquisition. Offshore manufacturing of prosthetic components may help hold down costs, but also threatens longer and more frequent problems with back-ordered components.

Challenges for the future

There are numerous interesting areas for near-term progress in the arena of lower extremity prosthetics. The research being done at Northwestern University by Childress' group regarding rollover shape offers the first new insight into prosthetic alignment in generations [2]. It holds the potential to turn the alignment process into a scientific procedure and probably one that can be automated. The amount of time that could be saved compared with today's trial-and-error process is difficult to imagine.

Measurement technology is another area where tremendous improvements in understanding of the process offer to alter radically the ability to obtain consistently the desired result of a comfortable and stable fit. New limb measurement technologies offer to collect data not only about limb volume and contours, but also regarding tissue density, vascular supply, and precise location of internal structures, such as scars and neuromas. New measurement technologies also apply to outcomes measurement. No consistent protocol has yet been adopted for use in the documentation and quantification of prosthetic outcomes. The need for change in this area is driven by managed care and the need to provide a rationale for the medical necessity of components and designs prescribed and fitted. Without an accepted outcomes assessment protocol, the prosthetic profession will remain vulnerable to arbitrary decisions and denials at the hands of case managers who lack basic knowledge of the field.

The next three decades promise to challenge the prosthetic profession greatly as it is now constituted. The leading edge of the baby boom is approaching retirement age and soon will need increasing medical care, including prosthetic care. Add the population growth to the increasing percentage of obese and diabetic individuals in the population, and the need for an increasing number of skilled prosthetists in the future is clear. Unless new technologies can be harnessed to accelerate the fitting process, or new ways can be found to recruit and train prosthetists more rapidly, the profession faces a frightening manpower shortage. Only the identification of a cure for diabetes could prevent the need from exceeding the supply.

It may not make much of a difference in the manpower shortage, but the presence of two new schools offering advanced degrees in orthotics and prosthetics is a significant step in the professionalization of the field (eg, MSPO Program, School of Applied Physiology, Georgia Institute of Technology, Atlanta, Georgia; Eastern Michigan University, Ypsilanti, Michigan). These more academically trained professionals will bring into the field the research skills that prosthetists have long lacked. Hope runs high that these new professionals will lead the way in addressing the above-identified problems.

References

[1] M. Marriott Robo legs. New York Times. Monday June 20, 2005:E1, 8.
[2] Hansen AH, Childress DS, Knox EH. Prosthetic foot roll-over shapes with implications for alignment of transtibial prostheses. Prosthet Orthot Int 2000;24:205–15.

ELSEVIER
SAUNDERS

Phys Med Rehabil Clin N Am
17 (2006) 31–48

PHYSICAL MEDICINE
AND REHABILITATION
CLINICS OF
NORTH AMERICA

Lower Extremity Socket Design and Suspension

Kevin Carroll, MS, CP, FAAOP

*Hanger Prosthetics & Orthotics, Hanger Orthopedic Group, Inc.,
Orlando, FL, USA*

Transtibial and transfemoral socket design

The socket is the crucial first component of any lower extremity prosthesis. Being in direct contact with an individual's residual limb makes the socket an extension of the body. The fit and comfort of the socket usually determine whether or not the individual wears the prosthesis. Systems for transtibial, transfemoral, and hip disarticulation and hemipelvectomy (HD/HP) sockets have undergone dramatic improvements in recent years. New materials, such as urethanes, mineral-based liners, and improved silicones, are much more flexible than the hard plastics that were used for decades. *Memory* is the term prosthetists use to describe the responsiveness of the socket material. Memory is what enables the socket to change shape as an individual moves. When stepping forward, the socket expands to accommodate the enlargement of the muscles, then instantly contracts when the muscles relax in the swing phase of the gait. These dynamic materials also are gentle against the underlying skin.

Comparing a dynamic socket with one fabricated in the 1980s or early 1990s shows a striking visual difference. The dynamic socket is uniquely contoured and flexible to the touch, whereas older styles were fabricated from hard, rigid materials. Prosthetists now have a greater understanding of the underlying anatomy of the residual limb, allowing them to surface match the socket interface to the residual limb. This ability is of particular relevance in casting or scanning transtibial and transfemoral sockets. When the muscles, bony prominences, and vascular structure of the residual limb are individually mapped, the result is a custom-fit socket that is contoured to match the unique limb. The socket's anatomically correct shape allows for total surface contact with the residual limb; this leads

E-mail address: kcarroll@hanger.com

1047-9651/06/$ - see front matter © 2006 Elsevier Inc. All rights reserved.
doi:10.1016/j.pmr.2005.11.001

to even distribution of weight across the surface, rather than concentrated pressure points, as seen in older lower extremity designs. The user's muscles fire comfortably into the specific channels that have been built into the socket. For added stability, the socket sits inside a semirigid carbon fiber frame. Specific areas of the frame are trimmed out to maintain the flexibility and comfort of the socket.

The expansion and contraction capability of the total contact socket massages the residual limb and is particularly beneficial for dysvascular amputees. Venous return is increased, and swelling, pain, and discomfort are reduced. The socket's direct contact with the skin also provides greater sensory feedback to the user. Older adults are able to have more control of their prosthesis without the risk of causing damage to the fragile skin of their residual limb.

Many researchers are focusing on the benefits of precisely mapping the vascular and nerve structures of the residual limb. Symptoms such as numbness in the residual limb and excessive fatigue after wearing the prosthesis a few hours may indicate pressure hot spots where the socket is restricting circulation or pressing on nerves. Better mapping of the residual limb is the key to eliminating these problems. Research also has yielded the introduction of computer scanning systems into the socket fabrication process. The prosthetist can begin the fitting process by scanning the individual's residual limb with a laser scanner or wand. This scanning captures an exact three-dimensional computer image of the limb and relays it to an automated carver, which shapes the socket precisely (Fig. 1).

The socket is the foundation for the lower extremity prosthetic user's comfort. Pain is not a mandatory part of wearing a prosthesis, even though many

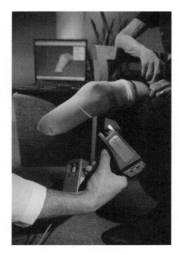

Fig. 1. Computerized scanning systems such as Hanger's Insignia make the prosthetic fitting process easier and more accurate. (Courtesy of Hanger Prosthetics & Orthotics; with permission.)

users have been told otherwise. Pain indicates a problem that needs to be analyzed and corrected. By understanding the overriding importance of the socket's shape and fit, prosthetic users, their physicians, and their therapists are much more likely to achieve success in the rehabilitation process.

Transtibial sockets

In addition to the total contact socket described previously, there are a few older variations of transtibial sockets that are still commonly in use. The patellar tendon bearing socket has an anterior wall that extends over a portion of the patella [1]. A contour that is built in below the patella is a unique design feature that allows for weight bearing on the patellar ligament. The posterior wall helps keep the ligament positioned against the contour by applying a counterforce. This design can lead to problems of skin breakdown at the patella ligament for some users.

Individuals with short residual limbs may prefer a supracondylar/suprapatellar socket that features higher medial, lateral, and anterior walls. A contour is built into the socket proximal to the patella, and the socket extends over the entire patella and femoral condyles [1]. Some advantages of this design are better knee stability, added suspension, and a larger surface area for weight bearing.

Another option for transtibial users is the suction socket. A silicone liner offers the advantages of reducing friction on the skin during walking. It also provides suction between the skin and the silicone that keeps the socket suspended. This liner provides a level of cushioning that is far superior to older Pelite and leather liners.

Transfemoral sockets: historical perspective

Historically, the transfemoral prosthesis has presented more challenges than the transtibial prosthesis in terms of design and use. The higher point of amputation and the absence of the natural knee joint also make alignment more difficult. The challenges that are inherent in transfemoral sockets are reflected by a more extensive history of development and research.

The quadrilateral socket, a squared-off design, was the most commonly worn transfemoral socket from the 1950s through the 1980s. The goal of fitting the quadrilateral socket was to position the ischial tuberosity on the outside edge of the socket and to ensure the tuberosity did not work its way gradually inside the socket. In evaluations of quadrilateral socket users around the world, the author has observed thousands of cases in which the tuberosity was inside the socket, creating a much better socket fit. During ambulation, the usual lateral shifting of the socket away from the body was eliminated. The improvement in gait was offset by a painful pressure hot spot where the socket touched the ramus bone. By lowering the medial wall, this pressure was relieved, whereas anterior/posterior pressure built into the socket kept the user from sinking too low in the socket.

The first major shift away from the quadrilateral socket came when prosthetist Ivan Long introduced the normal shape–normal alignment socket in the late 1970s. This design is based on a medial-to-lateral fit that is tight without causing pressure and discomfort on the soft tissues. When the user stands on the prosthesis, he or she has excellent medial-lateral control, resulting in excellent alignment when walking. The femur of the residual limb is held in an anatomically correct position that matches the alignment of the sound femur [2]. Long believed that if the medial-lateral dimension was correct, ischial containment was unnecessary. One disadvantage for some users with soft tissue is that when the user is seated, the anterior aspect sticks up considerably above that of the sound leg. Although this socket worked well when Long—a master prosthetist—was fitting it, some other prosthetists have had difficulty in achieving a successful fit.

In the early 1980s, prosthetist John Sabolich introduced a socket called contoured adducted trochanteric–controlled alignment method. This socket attempts to lock the ischial tuberosity bone into the socket to prevent lateral shifting. Ischial containment continues to be a key technique in transfemoral socket design. Weight bearing in the ischial containment socket is focused mainly through the medial aspect of the ischium and the ischial ramus [3].

The ischium and ramus are centered firmly against the posterior aspect of the socket, and pressure distribution occurs across the surface of the residual limb [4,5]. Additional weight bearing comes from the gluteal muscles. To address the problem of anterior gapping of the socket when the user sat down, Sabolich added a flexible posterior wall to the design. Noting that gradual volume loss in the residual limb caused the user to "sink" down into the socket, the medial wall was trimmed lower to eliminate a pressure hot spot. Later, the contoured Sabolich socket was introduced; this design gave some users more stability.

In the 1980s, the author worked with a group of clinicians doing anatomic research at the University of Oklahoma and Oklahoma State University. Analysis and dissection of human cadavers increased understanding of muscle structure and function in the residual limb, particularly in the area of how to create hypertrophy of the muscles versus atrophy by applying pressure between the muscles. One conclusion was that the fatty tissue of the ischial rectal fascia could cushion the tuberosity bone if the socket could contain the tissue. Aggressive ischial-ramus containment sockets were doing just the opposite, however—squeezing the fatty tissue out of the socket and causing bony pressure points. By accommodating the tissue inside the socket, it was discovered that users could stand and sit on a natural cushion of their soft fatty tissue. With detailed analysis of the human anatomic structure, the author's group also questioned if ischial containment was truly an achievable goal. By measuring 50 human skeletons, it was determined that the average distance from the tuberosity bone to the ischial spine was $1\frac{3}{4}$ inches. When the socket's medial containment of the ischial ramus extends further than $1\frac{3}{4}$ inches, the user experiences painful pressure hot spots on the sacrial tuberous and sacral spinous ligaments. It was concluded that true ischial containment sockets rarely exceed $1\frac{3}{4}$ inches of containment of the ischial-ramus, and are most effective in cases of very short residual limbs. In cases in which it appears that a socket has more than $1\frac{3}{4}$ inches of containment, what has actually happened is that the socket has rotated away from the ligaments, and the ischial ramus is not contained at all (Fig. 2) [6].

Dynamic transfemoral sockets

The highly contoured flexible sockets favored by transfemoral users today are a direct result of ongoing research. MRI and CT scans have provided a window into the dynamic world of muscle function in the residual limb. Changes in the shape of the muscles are clearly visible as living research subjects alternately contract and relax their thighs. It is reasonable to conclude that, ideally, the socket also should have a changing and dynamic nature. When the socket is fabricated from a rigid material, and the individual actively fires the muscle when walking, it pushes painfully against the hard socket wall, sending a basic message to the user's brain: "Stop firing the muscle." In just a few weeks, the muscle is atrophied. Conversely, a dynamic socket allows the muscle to fire freely into its own compartment within the socket. The muscle quickly becomes vital and strong—hypertrophied (Fig. 3).

The design of the dynamic transfemoral socket combines a thin, bioelastic socket with a supportive outer frame composed of composite materials. Key areas of the frame are cutout to allow for painless expansion of the

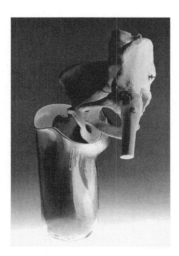

Fig. 2. Ischial containment sockets for above-knee prosthetic users capture the ischium and ramus bones within the socket. This increases stability and comfort. (Courtesy of Hanger Prosthetics & Orthotics; with permission.)

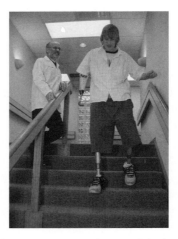

Fig. 3. Dynamic socket design encourages muscle strength in the residual limb, increasing an individual's mobility. (Courtesy of Hanger Prosthetics & Orthotics; with permission.)

muscles during stance phase. The responsive material instantly clamps back onto the limb as the muscles relax during swing phase. From the first time they don their dynamic prosthesis, transfemoral users are taught to fire their muscles actively and use them every time they walk. Ideally, the residual limb is in direct contact with the socket—no gel liners or socks in between. This direct contact enables the user to feel the prosthesis, increasing his or her control and proprioception (Fig. 4).

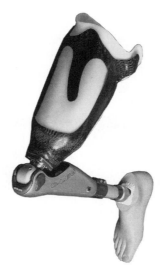

Fig. 4. The dynamic transfemoral socket sits inside a supportive frame; cutouts allow for expansion of the muscles. (Courtesy of Hanger Prosthetics & Orthotics; with permission.)

Although walking comfort is important, the average individual spends more time sitting down, so how the socket feels when sitting also is of concern. On dynamic sockets, the flexible posterior wall relaxes under the weight of the residual limb and upper body. A corresponding cutout in the composite frame allows for further socket expansion and comfort when sitting. Transfemoral users should be encouraged to sit down in their socket frequently as they are being fitted and to ask for modifications as needed to increase comfort (Fig. 5).

With the routine use of test sockets and new computer scanning techniques, the fitting process for transfemoral users has been greatly improved. A test socket is similar to a rough draft of a written document. The prosthetist and the patient have the opportunity to make many small and large modifications. Contouring, trim lines, and placement of cutouts on the outer frame are some of the socket features that are carefully planned and modified. The ultimate result is a truly customized final definitive socket (Fig. 6).

Suspension: transtibial and transfemoral

Not every transtibial or transfemoral user is a good candidate for a direct suction socket. Limiting factors may include the individual's general state of health; the presence of bony prominences, skin problems, or other issues with the residual limb; or a very short residual limb. Numerous other suspension options are available.

Many prosthetic users wear suspension sleeves as either a primary or a secondary means of suspension. The sleeve is rolled on over the prosthesis, extending for several inches above the knee. It makes direct contact with the skin on the user's thigh, sealing off the top of the socket to prevent air from entering. Sleeves are easy and effective to use. The synthetic material is vulnerable to punctures, making it necessary to replace sleeves regularly. Sleeves are meant to be airtight and as such can cause problems with perspiration and discomfort for individuals who live in hot or humid areas. Prescription and

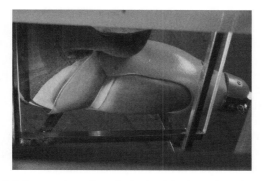

Fig. 5. This clear chair bottom shows how the back of the dynamic socket relaxes when the individual sits down. (Courtesy of Hanger Prosthetics & Orthotics; with permission.)

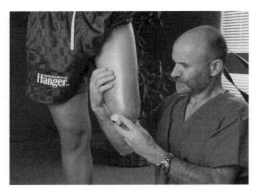

Fig. 6. Test sockets allow the prosthetist to make modifications and achieve an ideal fit for each individual. (Courtesy of Hanger Prosthetics & Orthotics; with permission.)

over-the-counter antiperspirants are available to help reduce perspiration. The latest generation of suspension sleeves incorporates a simple valve into the sleeve. Any air that pushes up out of the top of the socket during ambulation or when the user sits down or stands up is released through the valve.

Gel liners introduce suction and tackiness between the skin and the liner and can provide primary or secondary suspension for the prosthesis [7]. Gel liners also add a cushioning, protective layer when the residual limb has scar tissue, skin grafts, or bony prominences. Gel liners with a pin-lock system greatly reduce the odds of individuals losing the prosthesis as they move through their day. The liner is rolled onto the residual limb and has a pin extending from the bottom of it that snaps into a lock in the bottom of the socket. It takes some practice for new users to learn to position the liner to hit the pin lock. Gel liners with pins pull heavily on the distal end of the residual limb and should not be used if there are distal invaginated areas [6]. Gel liners also are available with a lanyard system instead of a pin. A cord extends from the bottom of the gel liner and threads out through a hole at the end of the socket. The residual limb is simply pulled into the socket with the lanyard cord, and the cord is locked into place (Fig. 7).

Gel liners continue to evolve in new and innovative ways. One example is a gel liner that is worn in combination with a socket that has a valve positioned on the distal end. When the user dons the prosthesis, the air inside the socket is pushed out the valve, and as the individual walks, air continues to be pushed out the valve. The top of the socket is sealed by a sleeve that extends over the knee.

Gel liners with a built-in hypobaric silicone ring allow for suction suspension without the use of an external sleeve. A raised ring is positioned near the distal end of the liner, conforming to the shape of the internal socket wall and providing an airtight seal. When the user dons the prosthesis, air is pushed out through a distal valve, creating suction below the seal.

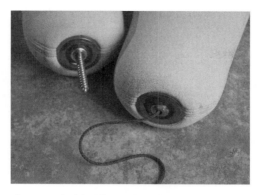

Fig. 7. Gel liners can be secured with either a pin lock or a lanyard system. Gel liners provide suspension while increasing comfort. (Courtesy of Hanger Prosthetics & Orthotics; with permission.)

Gel liners have many advantages. Anything that comes between the residual limb and the socket reduces proprioception, however, and the user's sense of control over the prosthesis. A useful comparison is wearing thin gloves versus thick gloves. It is much easier for an individual to feel what he or she is touching through a thin glove. For the same reason, it is a good idea to go with the thinnest gel liner possible that still provides the protective cushioning required by the individual (Fig. 8).

A vacuum-assisted suspension system (VASS) comprises a liner, suspension sleeve, and air evacuation pump. The concept behind VASS is to regulate volume fluctuations in the residual limb by creating an elevated vacuum between the liner and the socket wall. The vacuum pump may help reduce perspiration between the liner and the user's skin (Fig. 9).

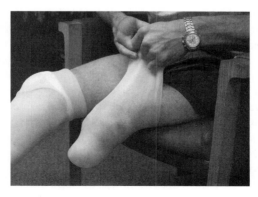

Fig. 8. Gel liners are soft and stretchy; a thinner liner enables the user to have better proprioception. (Courtesy of Hanger Prosthetics & Orthotics; with permission.)

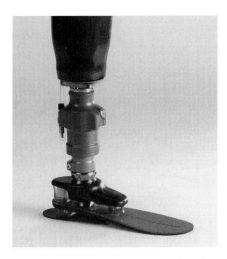

Fig. 9. The vacuum portion of VASS promotes natural fluid exchange that regulates volume fluctuation in the residual limb. (Courtesy of Hanger Prosthetics & Orthotics; with permission.)

For transfemoral users, the process of sitting down and standing up can cause concerns with suspension of the socket. A typical suction socket provides total contact between the residual limb and the socket. When the individual sits down or stands back up, there is a vulnerability to gaps between the socket and the residual limb, which can result in a loss of suction. If the user actively fires the muscles when he or she starts to sit down or stand back up, however, he or she has a much better chance of maintaining suction and keeping the prosthesis on. As discussed previously, the user must be taught from the beginning to be proactive in using and strengthening the thigh muscles. This skill comes into play in many areas of daily life, including getting into and out of a car and participating in sports and recreational activities.

Some individuals like to use a soft suspension belt for either primary or secondary suspension. The Silesian belt attaches to the socket on the lateral proximal wall and anterior medial wall and loops around the user's waist and opposite iliac crest. The belt is a simple and effective means of suspension; it should be removed and washed regularly or, if made of leather, replaced as needed to retain good hygiene. Another option is the total elastic suspension belt or Power Belt (Knit-Rite, Kansas City, Kansas). An elastic band wraps around the proximal 8 inches of the socket, then extends up the anterior and posterior aspect of the hip to form a belt that goes around the waist and fastens with Velcro [4]. These comfortable, flexible belts also enhance the user's rotational control of the prosthesis.

Older types of suspension are still in use. A thigh corset with metal joints that attach to the socket, a leather waist belt with a strap that buckles onto the socket (transtibial users), or a cuff strap around the knee (transtibial users) are a few examples. Newer modes of suspension are usually preferable, although there are individual situations in which an older suspension system works well.

Donning techniques for transfemoral users

Putting on a prosthesis, or donning, can be frustrating for many transfemoral users. Proper donning is important to maintain the suspension of the socket. Pulling the leg on while working the residual limb down into the socket can take a lot of energy. Older adults and individuals with diabetes are often lacking in upper body strength, and repeated gripping and pulling with their hands can result in injuries such as carpal tunnel syndrome or low back strain. Although there are many ways to don a suction socket, physicians and therapists should be familiar with the following four techniques.

One approach is to use a cotton sock that is pulled over the residual limb. The limb is worked down into the socket with a slight pumping action, and the sock is pulled out through the suction valve at the bottom of the socket. This approach to donning is common, but it is not particularly easy. Another option is known as the "wet fit." Lotion or liquid body powder is applied to the residual limb and the inside of the socket. This lotion reduces the friction of the skin against the socket, allowing the limb to slip down into place. Using an Ace bandage to aid in donning is another approach. Rather than wrapping it around the limb, the bandage is laid flat along the medial wall of the socket with the end of the bandage extending out the suction valve hole at the bottom of the socket. A slight pumping motion while rotating the bandage around the proximal edge works the residual limb and soft tissue into the socket as the Ace bandage is pulled gently through the suction valve hole. This pulls the tissue at the top of the limb down into the socket. This technique requires minimal strength and becomes even easier if lotion is used along with the bandage. Finally, the use of a nylon slip sock made of parachute material is another simple method. This thin, slippery sock is inverted into itself, then placed over the residual limb. After the limb has been worked down into the socket, the nylon slip sock is pulled out through the suction valve hole. There is no need for lotion or powder, making this a clean and simple donning method (Fig. 10).

Some individuals may have so much soft tissue they cannot pull all of it into the socket using the Ace bandage or the nylon slip sock alone. If soft tissues are lapping out the top of the socket after donning, the user should try combining these two donning techniques in the following manner: First, the individual unrolls an Ace bandage and lays it flat along the medial wall of the socket with the end of the bandage extending out the suction valve hole. Next, the individual places the inverted nylon slip sock over the residual limb and uses a slight pumping motion to work the limb down into the socket. Holding onto the top of the Ace bandage with one hand, the individual pulls the slip sock out through the valve hole, then gently pulls out the Ace bandage.

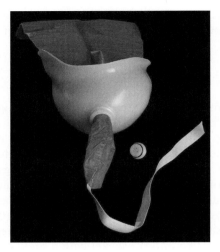

Fig. 10. Nylon slip socks can make it easier for some users to don their prosthesis. (Courtesy of Hanger Prosthetics & Orthotics; with permission.)

Hip disarticulation and hemipelvectomy socket design

Individuals who experience leg amputation at the level of HD or HP face tremendous challenges in their pursuit of mobility. In the absence of the natural ankle, knee, and hip joints, these high-level prosthetic users must expend 200% as much energy when walking as is required for normal ambulation [8,9]. Issues of comfort, control, balance, and stability all are magnified. Some HD/HP amputees are discouraged from even investigating the possibility of prosthetic care by well-meaning health care professionals. For individuals who do pursue the use of a prosthesis, research indicates that the highest rate of rejection of a prosthesis occurs among HD/HP users [10]. The primary cause of rejection is a poorly fitting socket that is uncomfortable. It has taken many years for HD/HP socket design to improve to the point where it is possible to achieve comfort and function.

Historical perspective

The tilting table prosthesis was introduced in the 1940s and was one of the first socket designs that addressed the specific needs of HD/HP users. The center of gravity was positioned through the hip joint, and to obtain stability, the hip was in a locked position. In the 1950s, McLaurin introduced the Canadian hip disarticulation prosthesis. The nonlocking hip joint was moved to the anterior, resulting in a smoother gait. The center of gravity was posterior to the hip joint and anterior to the knee joint during weight bearing, preventing the prosthesis from collapsing at the knee and hip [11,12]. Danish prosthetist Lynquist [13] designed a hip joint with 5° of pelvic tilt, making it possible for the ankle to move laterally. His design also had the stable anterior positioning of the hip joint. Lynquist [14] extended his work to encompass the needs of HP amputees, outlining a fitting process for "a Canadian-type plastic socket for hemi-pelvectomy." In 1957, Radcliffe [15] used science to validate McLaurin's approach to alignment of the prosthesis. Radcliffe's article, "The Biomechanics of the Canadian-Type Hip-Disarticulation Prosthesis" [15], supported the idea of shifting the center of gravity to fall posterior to the hip and anterior to the knee, an approach that continues as the alignment standard for today's HD/HP designs.

In the early 1980s, the author began fitting patients with an anatomically correct HD/HP socket. The mechanical hip joint was moved to the lateral aspect of the tuberosity as close to the acetabulum as possible, out-setting the hip joint in its own compartment within the socket and positioning it in the space previously occupied by the natural hip [16]. The author has witnessed a substantially higher rate of user acceptance with the anatomically correct socket. Results continue to develop as the author evaluates approximately 40 HD users and 20 HP users each year (Fig. 11).

Anatomically correct socket

The casting or scanning process for high-level anatomically correct sockets involves shaping the socket and capturing accurate anatomic details. Special definition is given to the suprailiac region, which the socket wraps around completely, improving suspension and reducing side-to-side pistoning. In an approach similar to the transfemoral suction socket, the HD prosthesis is suspended by containing the residual soft tissues within the socket [5,17]. In contrast to some previous HD/HP designs, this socket has a solid floor that is parallel to the ground, preventing the soft tissue from slipping

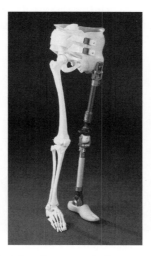

Fig. 11. By out-setting the hip joint, the anatomically correct HD/HP socket increases the user's stability and function. (Courtesy of Hanger Prosthetics & Orthotics; with permission.)

out of the socket as the user walks and moves about [16]. The author sees several cases of fractured ribs each year among users who have slipped through their socket; this occurs most frequently among postmenopausal women. When users feel like they may be slipping through, they tend to tighten the top of the socket, adding pressure beneath the rib cage and increasing the likelihood of a fracture (Fig. 12).

Ischial containment is a key concept in fitting HD sockets. Ischial containment stabilizes the medial-lateral and anterior-posterior aspects of the prosthesis, increases the user's control, and keeps the tuberosity inside the socket [18]. Lightweight thermoplastics are used to create the socket. and flexible areas are built-in to prevent painful hot spots of pressure [19]. Cushioning material can be used underneath the ischial tuberosity to relieve pressure. It is crucial to understand that the medial trim line of the socket cannot put pressure on the ramus. Pressure here guarantees pain for the user, and pain usually guarantees that the prosthesis will not be worn.

For HP users, capturing the sound buttock and a slight piece of the tuberosity within the socket increases the sense of control. This is easier said than done: 99% of the HP cases the author evaluates each year do not contain the ischial tuberosity on the sound side. The solution to this challenge is to capture the gluteal ring when casting or scanning the patient. The gluteal ring passes through the perineum, following the proximal area of Scarpa's triangle, then going lateral and inferior to the trochanter, returning to the inferior border of the gluteals. The gluteal muscles on the sound side are held within the socket during stance phase on the prosthesis, absorbing pressure [6].

The anatomically correct HD/HP socket allows for the thigh section to be even in length to the sound side. Also, the user's sound knee is level with the prosthetic knee when the user is sitting down. Some HD sockets position the hip component beneath the tuberosity, which causes the pelvis to tilt unnaturally while sitting and places pressure on the vertebrae, which can

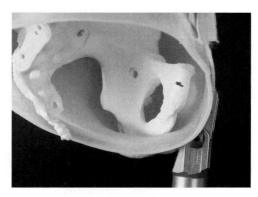

Fig. 12. This photo of bone placement within the anatomically correct HD/HP socket shows ischial containment and the solid socket floor under the residuum. (Courtesy of Hanger Prosthetics & Orthotics; with permission.)

lead to back pain and scoliosis. HD and HP users also report greater comfort when sitting with the anatomically correct socket because its design provides a level sitting surface for the tuberosities.

Unique considerations for hip disarticulation and hemipelvectomy

Some individuals choose not to use a prosthesis for ambulation. In these cases, the use of a specially designed "sitting socket" is crucial. Surgical disruption of the normal musculoskeletal attachments, combined with the effects of gravity over time, often lead to the development of scoliosis. Because HP amputees have lost half the muscle and tendon attachments that held the back straight, they are particularly vulnerable to scoliosis [16]. HD users are able to sit, stand, and walk in a more anatomically correct fashion, but still can develop scoliosis over time. Although scoliosis cannot be corrected completely, if it is detected early it is possible to keep it from worsening. HD/HP amputees should be examined carefully for scoliosis at least once a year. Sitting sockets are effective in reducing the tendency toward scoliosis and back alignment problems [20]. They also provide symmetric pressure distribution over the remaining ischial tuberosity. In some cases, it may be necessary to add an orthotic back brace; this is of particular importance if the individual uses a wheelchair part or all of the time. Sitting sockets also are recommended as a protective measure when HD/HP users participate in sporting activities in which a prosthesis is not worn. In cases of bilateral HD/HP, a sitting socket is essential to provide the individual with a stable sitting surface [16].

Just as some HD/HP users are discouraged from using a prosthesis, female users may be cautioned against becoming pregnant [21]. It is easy to see why the absence of a hip, or a hip and pelvic bone, might make it more difficult for a woman to carry a fetus during pregnancy; however, many HD/HP users have had normal pregnancies and normal vaginal deliveries. Because HD users still have the supportive bone structure of the pelvis, their bodies can support the weight of a pregnant uterus. As pregnancy progresses, and the size of the abdomen increases, the socket can be modified. Having lost one side of the pelvic structure, HP users may experience a dropped or tilted uterus. The author recommends that pregnant women take off their prosthesis at 20 weeks' gestation to eliminate placing undue pressure on the growing fetus. Some women prefer to stop wearing their prosthesis earlier in their pregnancy. A supportive maternity sling that extends under the abdomen can be helpful.

Suspension: hip disarticulation and hemipelvectomy

The upper and lower trim lines of the socket have a critical effect on the function and comfort of the limb. Because the HD socket is suspended by locking onto the user's torso just above the iliac crests, the upper trim line is usually just above the iliac crests [16]. By extending it an inch or so higher, however, weight bearing is distributed over a larger area, making it easier to walk. In cases of HP amputation, because the individual no longer has an iliac crest, the soft tissues are being compressed and shaped to achieve adequate suspension, and the upper trim line should extend even higher above the waist. Bringing it up to the ribcage provides additional support for the back and may act as a brace to reduce scoliosis. These higher trim lines must be tempered, however, to allow for movement and bending at the waist. The lower anterior edge of the HP socket often extends down so far that it may push into the user's proximal thigh section when he or she sits down; this causes some discomfort, but the benefit is that it maintains a counterforce in the direction of the tuberosity and gluteals. Ultimately, the individual must understand that trimming out the socket is a compromise. What may be lost in terms of comfort improves the limb in terms of function, or some function may be sacrificed to improve comfort [6].

For individuals with tissue breakdown or other problems on the residuum, it is a good idea to add a low-modulus, gel-type liner under the socket. The best way to do this is to modify a large gel liner by cutting a hole for the sound leg to go through [16]. The liner is stretched up around the user's trunk, adding a protective layer between the skin and the socket. Another option is to have a custom gel liner made by a prosthetist. Friction on the soft tissues is reduced, and the low-modulus material provides a more even distribution of pressure [18]. Liners reduce abrasions and increase comfort, enabling individuals to wear their prostheses for longer periods.

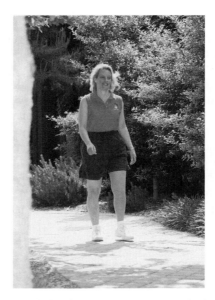

Fig. 13. New prosthetic technologies allow lower extremity prosthetic users to lead active lives. (Courtesy of Hanger Prosthetics & Orthotics; with permission.)

Summary

The availability of advanced materials and techniques means that lower extremity prosthetic users of all ages and amputation levels can achieve a more complete lifestyle recovery. The key component of any lower extremity prosthesis is the socket. The socket is the foundation for the user's comfort, and comfort is the foundation for restoring a individual's mobility. Dynamic sockets, "high-tech" liners, and individualized fitting practices are key elements in achieving comfort. Various available suspension systems address the needs of virtually all users. Finally, emerging technologies indicate an even brighter future for all individuals who use a lower extremity prosthesis (Fig. 13).

References

[1] Kapp S, Cummings D. Transtibial amputation: prosthetic management. In: American Academy of Orthopaedic Surgeons. Atlas of limb prosthetics. St Louis: CV Mosby; 1992. p. 453–78.

[2] Long I. Walking normally with an above knee prosthesis. In Motion 2003;13:18–20.

[3] Radcliffe CW. Comments on new concepts for above knee sockets. In: Donovan R, Pritham C, Wilson AB Jr, editors. Report of ISPO Workshops, International Workshop on Above-Knee Fitting and Alignment. Copenhagen: International Society for Prosthetics and Orthotics; 1989. p. 31–7.

[4] Schuch CM. Transfemoral amputation: prosthetic management. In: American Academy of Orthopaedic Surgeons. Atlas of limb prosthetics. St Louis: CV Mosby; 1992. p. 509–33.

[5] Sabolich J. Contoured adducted trochanteric-controlled alignment method: introduction and basic principles. Clin Prosthet Orthot 1985;9:15–26.

[6] Carroll K, Baird J, Binder K. Transfemoral prosthetic designs: prosthetics and patient management: a comprehensive clinical approach. Thorofare (NJ): SLACK Incorporated; 2006, in press.

[7] Uellendahl J. Prosthetic socks and liners. In: First step: a guide for adapting to limb loss. Knoxville (TN): National Limb Loss Information Center; 2001. p. 56–8.

[8] Huang CT. Energy cost of ambulation with Canadian hip disarticulation prosthesis. J Med Assoc Alabama 1983;52:47–8.

[9] Waters RL, Perry J, Antonelli C, Hislop H. Energy costs of walking of amputees: the influence of level of amputation. J Bone Joint Surg Am 1976;58:42–6.

[10] Jensen JS, Mandrup-Poulsen T. Success rate of prosthetic fitting after major amputations of the lower limb. Prosthet Orthot Int 1983;7:119–22.

[11] McLaurin CA. Hip disarticulation prosthesis. Report No. 15. Toronto: Prosthetic Services Center, Department of Veterans Affairs; 1954.

[12] McLaurin CA, Hampton F. Diagonal type socket for hip disarticulation amputees. Chicago: Northwestern University Prosthetic Research Center, Publication V.A.-V1005 M 1079; 1961.

[13] Lynquist E. New hip joint for Canadian-type hip disarticulation prosthesis. Artif Limbs 1958;4:129–30.

[14] Lynquist E. Canadian-type plastic socket for a hemi-pelvectomy. Artif Limbs 1958;5:130–2.

[15] Radcliffe CW. The biomechanics of the Canadian-type hip disarticulation prosthesis. Artif Limbs 1957;4:29–38.

[16] Carroll K. Hip disarticulation and transpelvic amputation: prosthetic management. In: Smith DG, Michael JW, Bowker JH, editors. Atlas of amputations and limb deficiencies: surgical, prosthetic, and rehabilitation principles. 3rd edition. Rosemont (IL): American Academy of Orthopaedic Surgeons; 2004. p. 565–73.

[17] Sabolich J, Guth T. The CAT-CAM-HD: a new design for hip disarticulation patients. Clin Prosthet Orthot 1988;12:119–22.

[18] Angelico J. Sockets for hip disarticulation and hemipelvectomy amputees. In Motion 2001;
     11:19–20.
[19] Imler C, Quigley M. A technique for thermoforming hip disarticulation prosthetic sockets.
     J Prosthet Orthot 1990;3:34–7.
[20] Stark G. Overview of hip disarticulation prostheses. Am Acad Orthot Prosthet 2001;13:
     50–3.
[21] Skoski CHP. HD HELP. Available at: www.hdhphelp.org. Accessed January 29, 2004.

ELSEVIER
SAUNDERS

Phys Med Rehabil Clin N Am
17 (2006) 49–72

PHYSICAL MEDICINE
AND REHABILITATION
CLINICS OF
NORTH AMERICA

Progressive Upper Limb Prosthetics

Chris Lake, CPO, FAAOP*, Robert Dodson, CPO

*Advanced Arm Dynamics of Texas, 3501 North Macarthur Boulevard, Suite 650,
Irving, TX 75062, USA*

The field of upper limb prosthetics has become increasingly specialized [1]. At the same time, most practitioners see few individuals with upper limb deficiency—typically one upper limb client per year compared with about 30 clients experiencing lower limb deficiencies. Within this relatively small number of upper limb deficiencies, practitioners rarely encounter what could be considered "common" mobility issues associated with lower limb prosthetics. In consideration of Dillingham et al's [2] findings, only 1908 of the approximately 18,496 annual upper limb deficiency cases involve styloid-level disarticulations to shoulder and interscapulothoracic levels. The other 16,588 individuals per year present with amputations distal to the wrist, which are much more difficult for a rehabilitation team to assess and treat.

This paradox of so few individuals needing such specialized care represents what prosthetists call the "upper extremity dilemma." It is extremely difficult for a large number of practitioners (approximately 3000 American Board of Certification in Orthotics and Prosthetics [ABC] Certified Prosthetists [CPs] and Certified Prosthetist/Orthotists [CPOs] [ABC, personal communication, August 2005]) to increase their upper extremity knowledge with such a small patient base [3]. In contrast, practitioners have much more success honing their lower extremity skills in even a moderately busy practice given the nearly 113,702 lower limb deficiencies per year (56,912 Syme's level and proximal).

Given the small number of patients and the highly technical aspects of upper limb prosthetics, upper limb treatment has earned its place as a specialty within the larger field of rehabilitation. Based on the Academy Upper Limb Society enrollment in summer 2005, approximately 66 individuals in the United States pursue upper limb prosthetics as a specialty. Some of these well-known specialists work for private companies that have upper limb specialty programs, whereas others have university-based and private practices.

---

* Corresponding author.
E-mail address: clake@armdynamics.com (C. Lake).

1047-9651/06/$ - see front matter © 2006 Elsevier Inc. All rights reserved.
doi:10.1016/j.pmr.2005.10.004
pmr.theclinics.com

This article provides readers with basic knowledge of progressive upper limb prosthetics. This knowledge is based on clinical protocols and the real-life cases presented by members of the Academy Certificate Course in Upper-Limb Prosthetics. Much of this information is presented in general concept summaries of larger topics. For more in-depth information on these topics, the reader is directed to the Further Readings and References.

Understanding the unique differences of upper limb deficiency

Beyond the obvious differences between the two distinct levels of deficiency, it is crucial to understand the unique nature of upper limb impairment [4]. Typically, an individual has little or no warning of the impending loss. Most upper limb amputations result from a traumatic event. Most patients experience no preoperative stage in which they can attempt to prepare for life after an amputation. In many cases, an individual wakes up in the recovery room to find that he or she has lost part or all of one or both upper extremities. He or she must grapple with the physical pain of the injury and amputation, while facing the psychological blow of feeling less capable and independent in a world that often measures self-worth by what an individual can do.

In addition, it is difficult to disguise the loss of an upper limb. Most social interaction centers on a person's face and torso, and even casual onlookers may notice the missing limb. In contrast, lower limb amputees have an easier time adapting into society. Unless these individuals are wearing shorts, their level of deficiency can go undetected for quite some time, giving them the opportunity to share their feelings, particularly in the early days, in a more comfortable and supportive setting.

Many upper limb amputees have extremely high expectations for what a prosthesis can accomplish. Today's media and films often exaggerate the technical aspects of upper limb prosthetics. Patients may come in envisioning futuristic devices. Although an upper limb electrical prosthesis can be very sophisticated, most are less advanced than what patients expect. Some of this difference involves complex biomechanical principles being replaced in the upper limb versus mostly mechanical and weight bearing principles being replaced in the lower limb. Range of motion, dexterity, and strength all play a role in upper limb functionality. At this time, it may not be possible to equal all pre-amputation physical abilities of a patient with current technology. The rehabilitation team should encourage patients to ask questions about the pros and cons of different prosthetic options. Similarly, it is helpful to inform clients of the latest in prosthetic research and what could be on the horizon in the near future for their prosthetic care.

Many patients balk at the suggestion of seeking counseling, but it is crucial to encourage clients to recognize the many complex feelings that can surround an upper limb deficiency. The sense of touch is a fundamental tool that humans use to convey feeling and emotion to each other. The loss of even portions of the fingers can challenge clients and make them feel isolated or lacking in a fundamental way. The human hand is a miraculous biologic achievement that allows its owner to engage in a multitude of activities, ranging from simply wearing a wedding ring to performing sophisticated job tasks. The greater the scope of the upper limb loss, the more deeply a patient may feel powerless and dependent. A carefully fitted prosthesis can return many important functions, but it also is essential that the individual's sense of loss be acknowledged and self-esteem be restored. In addition, psychological evaluation can provide insight on how patients learn. Knowing a client's unique personal learning style can help the clinician design the most successful training program.

Foundation

Progressive upper limb prosthetic care hinges on the initial patient assessment. The length of amputation, level of amputation, and prosthetic options all play a vital role in the ultimate patient outcome. The initial surgical and occupational therapy can be likened to the bedrock on which a stable house stands, whereas the initial assessment is similar to the piers that anchor and stabilize the house, elevating it to its maximum potential and functionality.

Surgical and therapeutic implications

The best type of surgical technique for an upper limb–deficient individual is a myodesis approach, in which the surgeon sutures the residual muscles to the bone rather than to one another. This technique creates a much more stable platform for all forms of prosthetic management. Muscles can contract independently without soliciting undesired movement in nearby muscles. This particular surgical technique also creates clean, independent muscle delineation in the myoelectric user.

Early identification and treatment of adherent scar tissue are important because these painful adhesions deprive patients of the full potential of their prosthesis (Fig. 1). Adherences can be skin to bone, skin and muscle to bone, or any combination thereof. These adherences cause pain when contracting muscles or extending the residual limb through the appropriate motions needed to operate a body-powered prosthesis. Adherent scar tissue should be treated early and aggressively; this may require surgical management and aggressive occupational therapy. Lack of occupational therapy may lead to the unnoticed progression of such adhesions. Before prosthetic management begins, the following crucial occupational therapy procedures need to be done:

- Wound care
- Scar management
- Soft tissue mobilization
- Residual limb shaping
- Range of motion therapy and general muscle strengthening
- Edema control

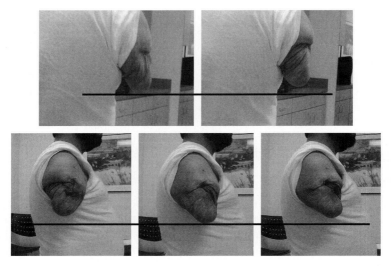

Fig. 1. Presentation of adherent scar tissue at the transhumeral level. Resting position (*top left*). On cocontraction of biceps and triceps (*top right*). Resting position (*bottom center*). Contraction of the triceps and biceps (*bottom left and right*).

Limb length plays an important role in what components can and cannot be fitted to the patient. Crucial decisions are made during surgery that can affect an amputee's prosthetic livelihood. In general, the longer the residual limb, the easier it is for patients to operate a body-powered or electrical prosthesis. The transradial level is usually the best scenario. With the preservation of the elbow, patients have an enhanced functional envelope, particularly when using an electrical prosthesis. For higher degrees of amputation, such as transhumeral and glenohumeral levels, an electrical prosthesis may prove to be a more functional option, secondary to the lack of excursion. Excursion requirements are based on harness anchor and reaction points that are determined by the length of the residual limb. High transhumeral and shoulder levels exhibit a 40% decrease in excursion ability compared with transradial levels [5]. Excessive limb length also can be problematic and limit the client's prosthetic choices. Another concern in this situation is that the prosthesis may look less "natural," which may make patients unhappy and less inclined to use the device.

Transcarpal styloid level considerations

The transcarpal styloid level allows for preservation of full supination, pronation, and wrist flexion and extension, provided that no traumatic event limits motion. Surgeons can make an anatomic decision about the styloids to enhance pronation and supination. Until more recently, prosthetists fitted these patients with passive prostheses. Now technologic advances with shortened electrical (transcarpal) hands combine functionality with a better esthetic appearance and bilateral length symmetry. The transcarpal hand also can be adapted to a quick disconnect wrist that allows amputees to switch back and forth between electrical terminal devices designed for specific tasks or more lifelike appearance (Fig. 2).

Transradial level considerations

The transradial level is the most common level of amputation seen by the prosthetist. In general, these amputees benefit from having a longer residual limb that better distributes force across their limb during daily activities. For optimal prosthetic component selection, the postoperative residual limb length, including distal soft tissues, should be at least 10 cm proximal to the ulnar styloid. This length allows for the greatest ease in body-powered and electrical component selection [6]. Conventional components, such as a five-function wrist and electrical components incorporating powered rotators, all fit comfortably, and this clearance accommodates cabling, wiring, and any necessary socket clearance (Fig. 3).

Elbow disarticulation considerations

Although suspension is optimal, and humeral rotation can be captured, this level is the least desirable because of cosmetic issues and limitation of applicable prosthetic elbows. Unless the patient needs an elbow that allows external/internal rotation, it is best to fit this type of limb with outside locking hinges. These hinges add at least 1 more inch of mediolateral dimension in the finished prosthesis. This increased clearance can create problems with the patient's clothing. Also, amputees often dislike the general appearance. Aside from these drawbacks, keeping the elbow joint intact results in superior weight bearing and force distribution (Fig. 4) [6].

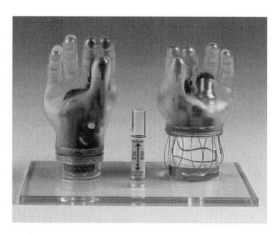

Fig. 2. Comparison of standard electric hand (*left*) and Otto Bock Transcarpal Hand (*right*). (Courtesy of Otto Bock, Minneapolis, MN.)

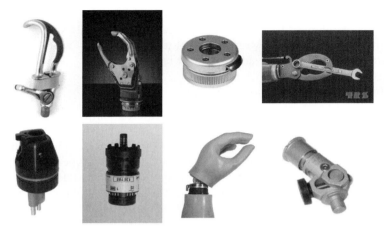

Fig. 3. Common prosthetic components at the transradial level include electrical and body-powered wrist rotators, terminal devices, and elbows. (Courtesy of Hosmer, Cambell, CA; Otto Bock, Minneapolis, MN; TRS, Boulder, CO; Texas Assistive Devices, Brazoria, TX; and Motion Control, Salt Lake City, UT.)

A surgical technique known as the Marquardt procedure can help patients maximize their mobility and overall physical appearance. This procedure has shown good results in adult cases. It involves an angular osteotomy, which recreates the bulbous end associated with the elbow disarticulation while shortening the residual limb [7,8]. Implantation of internal hardware to replicate the condyles is currently under investigation and may offer similar results [9].

Transhumeral level considerations

With the elbow joint absent, the length of the residual limb is a key factor in the fitting and ultimate success of a prosthesis. To allow enough clearance

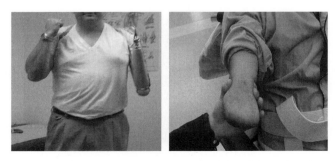

Fig. 4. The elbow disarticulation level can cause prosthetic length issues based on available elbow componentry, especially if prosthetic humeral rotation is required as seen in the picture on the left. The prominence of the condyles provides anatomic suspension and interface stability.

for the different types of conventional and electrical elbows, the postoperative residual limb, including distal soft tissue, should be at least 14 cm proximal to the most distal aspect of the olecranon. Cabling for internal elbow rotation locks for the conventional user and battery placement/wiring connections for the electrical user necessitate this amount of clearance (Fig. 5).

Glenohumeral and higher level considerations

Patients who have had cancer or severe trauma represent most amputations at the glenohumeral and higher levels (eg, interscapulothoracic). These cases involve unique issues and challenges. Their devices incorporate the greatest degree of prosthetic componentry, and it is crucial that the rehabilitation team exercise the utmost care in assessment and fitting. In particular, the team must respond promptly to common complications, such as prosthesis weight and heat dissipation (Fig. 6) [6].

Prosthetic options

Ideally, prosthetic options should be discussed during the initial patient assessment. It is important not to develop any preconceived notions as to what type of prosthesis a person requires or desires. The clinician's assumptions might be incorrect or at odds with a patient's recovery goals. Clinical

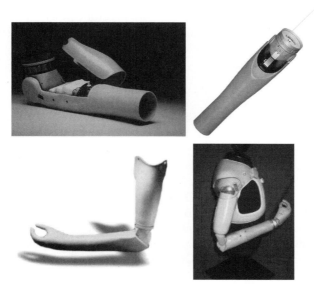

Fig. 5. Electrical and body-powered elbows for the transhumeral level. (Courtesy of Liberating Technologies, Inc., Holliston, MA; Otto Bock, Minneapolis, MN; and Motion Control, Salt Lake City, UT.)

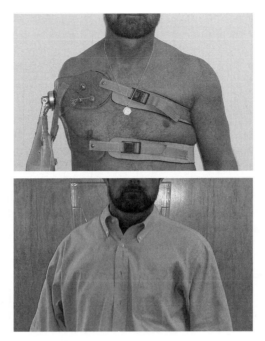

Fig. 6. By lowering the prosthetic shoulder joint, a better cosmesis is achieved.

experience shows that amputees eventually reject a prosthesis if it does not fulfill their basic personal requirements related to function, cosmetics, or psychological factors. Prosthetic options include the following:

- No prosthesis
- Passive prosthesis
- Body-powered prosthesis
- Electrically powered prosthesis
- Hybrid prosthesis
- Activity-specific prosthesis

No prosthesis

Many individuals decide not to wear a prosthesis for certain activities or choose not to wear one at all. Sometimes, a prosthesis does not significantly enhance the level of amputation, or the particular activity does not lend itself well to prosthetic enhancement. Other issues contributing to nonuse include poor initial prosthetic experience, discomfort from prosthetic design or weight, and lack of tactile sensation [10]. The acceptance and use of an upper limb prosthesis is enhanced dramatically when a patient is involved with an upper limb specialty program that incorporates expeditious prosthetic care and occupational therapy [11]. These two aspects are paramount in any successful specialty program.

One particular concern when choosing this option is the problem of overuse syndrome. Clinicians are just now beginning to understand the effects of overuse syndrome in individuals who do not wear a prosthesis or wear a particular type of prosthesis that does not provide them an optimal level of function. Overuse occurs in prosthetic users and individuals who have had a stroke and have essentially become one-handed [12,13]. Often, overuse can be found in the form of repetitive strain–type injuries in which the person uses poor body posture or ergonomics to address certain tasks. Any patient declining a prosthesis should be referred to an experienced occupational therapist. The therapist can show the amputee how to be one-handed and teach proper posture and ergonomics when working around the full range of motion of the body, especially above the head.

Passive prosthesis

A passive prosthesis closely mimics the contours and esthetics of a contralateral limb, but has no active type of grasping. Patients appreciate this design because its lightweight construction requires minimal harnessing and little maintenance. The passive prosthesis may incorporate hands that remain rigid, have positionable fingers, or have a spring-loaded passive type of grasping mechanism. These prostheses can be very functional, even though they are passive in design. Research has shown that prostheses that might be considered to be worn for purely cosmetic reasons are in fact used functionally when performing everyday tasks (Fig. 7) [14].

Body-powered prosthesis

Body-powered prostheses represent a common type of prosthesis fitted within the United States (Fig. 8). These body-powered devices are durable and often weigh less than their electrical counterparts. Their mechanics depend on proprioceptive feedback through the harness system. Disadvantages of a body-powered prosthesis revolve around the restrictive nature

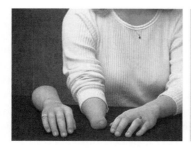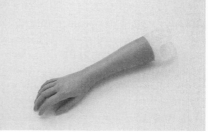

Fig. 7. Various passive prostheses. (Courtesy of ARTech Laboratory, Midlothian, TX.)

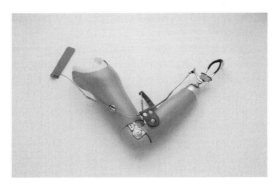

Fig. 8. Body-powered prosthesis.

of its design. The harness, which is required for functionality and suspension, limits the range of motion and functional envelope of the individual. (The *functional envelope* refers to the range of motion around a person's body in which he or she can operate the prosthesis without limiting or affecting the function of the contralateral limb.) When a patient uses a prosthesis outside the functional envelope, it becomes difficult to operate a terminal device without having to use gross body motion. These big-scale movements make it harder for amputees to use their intact side. As a result, they often rely on their intact side and do not use the prosthesis. Long-term use of a body-powered prosthesis can accelerate debilitating shoulder issues and anterior muscle imbalances and lead to nerve entrapment within the contralateral axilla [10,12,15].

Electrically powered prosthesis

The electrically powered prosthesis provides more grip force and enhanced functional envelope, while reducing or eliminating the overall harnessing necessary with a body-powered prosthesis. Many different designs are available. The term *myoelectric* commonly is associated with electrical prostheses even though other electrical control modalities exist. These include myoelectrodes, switches, slider-type input devices (servos, linear transducers, or potentiometers) and force-sensing resistors (or touch pads) [16].

1. *Myoelectrodes.* Myoelectrodes collect and filter surface electromyogram signals generated through muscle contractions and convert those signals into a form that can influence electrical motors (Fig. 9). Muscle sites are based primarily on the level of amputation and socket design and typically include the pectoralis, anterior deltoid, biceps, wrist flexors, posterior deltoid, infraspinatus, teres major, triceps, and wrist extensors. Any muscle that plays a reverse action or postural role should be evaluated carefully to avoid inadvertent and unwanted muscle contraction. A common example would be use of the trapezius for a myoelectric

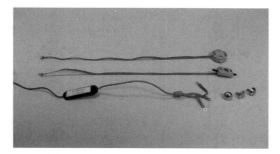

Fig. 9. Electrodes for the myoelectric prosthesis.

control site. Another area of concern is using a muscle for myoelectric control that is in close proximity to cardiac muscle, such as the pectoralis. A myoelectric site on this type of muscle could be affected by cardiac rhythm.

2. *Switch types*. A variety of motions are possible through different kinds of switching devices. Many switches are activated by pulling a cable or pressing a lever or button. Switches are designed to perform multiple functions and come in many presentations. Harness-type switches rely on excursion or some type of pull to actuate the switch. Depressing the switch with a chin, phocomelic finger, residual limb, or contralateral hand actuates another type of switch, often referred to as a push or "nudge" switch. A push switch may be placed distal to the axilla along the side of the torso or on the inner side of the person's forearm on a transradial level amputee and activated by humeral abduction. More advanced switches are found in multiposition types of applications. A typical multiposition switch might offer three positions. The first one is a resting position where no function occurs. The second position pronates the wrist upward. The third position rotates the wrist downward. In addition, switches can be momentary (providing brief actuation while the switch is activated) or latching (maintaining function until the person activates the switch again) (Fig. 10).

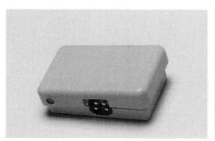
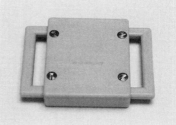

Fig. 10. Switches for the electrical prosthesis. (Courtesy of Otto Bock, Minneapolis, MN.)

3. *Slider-type input devices.* Slider-type input devices convert excursion distance, speed, or force into proportional movement of a prosthetic limb. As a result, feedback enhances proprioception as illustrated in the direct force or excursion relationship to elbow, wrist, or terminal device function (Fig. 11A). Slider-type actuators come in two varieties (Fig. 11B). The linear type of potentiometer is a Servo input device that translates linear motion or excursion into proportional function. Examples of this input device are the Liberating Technologies Linear Potentiometer (LTI, Inc., Holliston, MA) and Otto Bock's Linear Transducer (Otto Bock, Minneapolis, MN). The second variety is the force-sensing type of Servo such as Motion Control's ServoPro (Motion Control, Salt Lake City, UT). The force-sensing control translates information gathered via a strain gauge and interprets it to activate proportionally a device that has been preprogrammed through a microprocessor or electronic system. Both types of Servos provide increased proprioception through the association of force or linear pull (excursion) to proportional function. Although force-sensing Servos require less excursion, the amputee faces a fairly steep learning curve to master finite control. In contrast, a linear potentiometer depends on the simpler principles of excursion and gross body movement and is easier for most patients to master.

4. *Force-sensing resistors.* Some electrical prostheses employ a force-sensing resistor (Fig. 12). These types of input devices consist of a force-sensing resistor matrix, which interprets pressure in a proportional manner. The amputee activates the force-sensing resistor by moving the shoulder complex, a phocomelic finger, residual humeral neck, or other residual anatomy. These types of input devices represent a low-profile solution providing an inexpensive proportional input device. Special care in force-sensing resistor application into the prosthetic interface is crucial

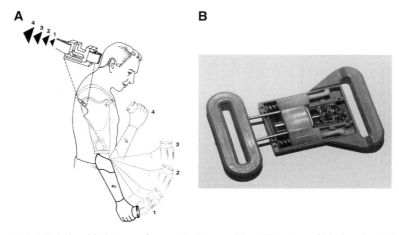

Fig. 11. (*A*) Relationship between force and elbow position. (Courtesy of Motion Control, Salt Lake City, UT.) (*B*) Otto Bock Linear Transducer. (Courtesy of Otto Bock, Minneapolis, MN.)

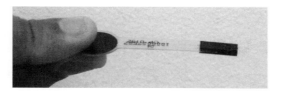

Fig. 12. Force-sensing resistors provide a low-profile, proportional input device.

to the success of the overall device. Improper installation results in premature failure and greater expense and can produce uncomfortable perspiration, moisture, and uneven shear force.

Myoelectric prostheses are a relatively new option, and with increased usage some exciting potential advantages are beginning to be seen. In particular, clinical experience is showing that myoelectric prostheses may prevent cortical reorganization and reduce the incidence of phantom pain [17]. In the authors' practice, patients who used a myoelectric prosthesis early in their rehabilitation reported less pain. Additional studies are needed to evaluate this phenomenon. It is important to discuss with the patient the different types of pain he or she may experience. The clinician also may need to explain that pain can take many forms, from the acute pain resulting from the surgical amputation itself to phantom pain and uncomfortable phantom sensations.

The chief drawback to an electrical prosthesis is its increased weight, which can cause muscle fatigue or friction about the residual limb. Moisture buildup also may pose a problem with electronic circuitry when proper fabrication techniques are not utilized. With the advent of water resistant terminal devices and electrodes, moisture is becoming less of an issue with the use of electronic prostheses.

There is a common misconception that body-powered prostheses are easier to maintain than electrical devices and require fewer repairs and overall maintenance. For the most part, clinical experience has debunked this myth. In reality, body-powered prostheses need maintenance just as frequently as electronic devices. Although it is true that it can cost more to repair an electronic prosthesis, downtime intervals tend to be similar or less than body-powered devices [18]. A proactive preventative maintenance program can greatly reduce overall patient frustrations with any prosthesis.

Hybrid prosthesis

The hybrid prosthesis combines the benefits of body-powered and electrical styles. This type of design allows simultaneous control of the elbow and terminal device and most commonly is simplified with the use of a body-powered elbow and electrical terminal device and wrist. In some cases, an amputee may choose a fully conventional system with an electronic wrist, but not

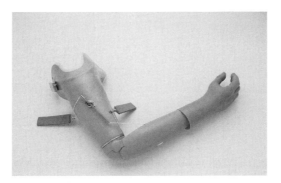

Fig. 13. Hybrid prosthesis.

usually as the first option. The previous discussion regarding body and externally powered prostheses is applicable to the hybrid-style prosthesis (Fig. 13).

Activity-specific prosthesis

The last prosthetic option is that of the activity-specific prosthesis. This type of prosthesis is designed for a specific activity where more typical prosthetic options are not sufficient. Patients in the authors' practice have used these custom devices successfully for activities such as gardening, weightlifting, and skydiving. The impact an activity-specific prosthesis can have on an amputee's overall quality of life cannot be overstated. These special prostheses allow patients to resume meaningful and exciting activities and help life "return to normal" in a tangible way. These devices also physically show to the amputee's family and friends that he or she is capable of doing many diverse activities (Fig. 14).

When discussing prosthetic options with patients, it is important to explore all the various options and work with patients to determine which approach best suits them and their needs. Often, more than one prosthesis is necessary to address all the patient's needs. With so many different types of prostheses now available, these devices should be viewed as valuable tools. Just as one would not want to limit his or her home toolbox to just a hammer or a screwdriver, an amputee should consider having several prosthetic "tools" to accomplish all the activities of daily living. Sometimes, one particular device can handle several kinds of activities. Other times, amputees are better served by using different types of terminal devices or an entirely different prosthesis.

Advances in upper limb technology

Current advances in upper limb technology can be divided into five categories:

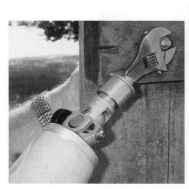
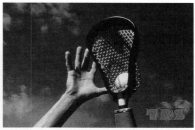
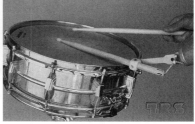

Fig. 14. Activity-specific terminal devices. (Courtesy of TRS, Boulder, CO; and Texas Assistive Devices, Brazonia, TX.)

- Treatment protocol
- Prosthetic interface
- Materials
- Microprocessor technology
- Terminal devices

Treatment protocol

Within the upper limb specialty clinic, treatment protocols revolve around the expedited delivery process. This process involves fitting the patient within 2 to 3 days, then following the patient consistently through occupational therapy. This close interaction allows clinicians to evaluate better the interface, component choice and use, and therapeutic issues. Patient frustration is reduced because problems can be identified quickly and alleviated. It has long been thought and shown that early return to function is optimal. In the 1980s, Malone et al [19] showed that individuals fitted within 30 days had higher rehabilitation success, returned to work earlier, and reported less pain from their amputation. In 2005, Fletchall [11], evaluating "the value of specialized rehabilitation of trauma and amputation," found similar trends indicating an approximate 96% success rate for patients who were seen immediately after their trauma versus a 56% success rate for those patients who were delayed from starting a specialized rehabilitation program. Additionally, 84% of those patients seen immediately by a specialized rehabilitation group remained in contact with their prosthetist/ therapist as compared to only 41% of those patients who were delayed from starting a specialized rehabilitation program. "This supports the theory that if an amputee receives therapy from a source that specializes, understands, fits him properly the first time, and trains him immediately, the amputee is going to retain the skill and knowledge for a longer period of time" [11].

During the expedited fitting process, the authors track patients closely through therapy. The rehabilitation team has found it helpful to use outcome and evaluation tools to determine progress. In addition, peer mentoring and interaction with other amputees helps patients adjust to their upper limb deficiency.

Prosthetic interface

A major determining factor of whether a patient will use a prosthesis comfortably is the design of prosthetic interface. In recent years, new techniques in socket interface design have been published. One type of interface method that has gained acceptance in lower limb prosthetics now is beginning to be used more frequently in upper limb prosthetics—the roll-on suction suspension liner. This design helps provide a positive type of suspension, while eliminating suspension harnessing, which allows the incorporation of more functional control harnessing. Roll-on liners can be used with all type of prostheses, including myoelectric prostheses (Fig. 15).

Flexible socket construction is a type of interface that enhances comfort through its flexibility, while allowing a more functional range of motion.

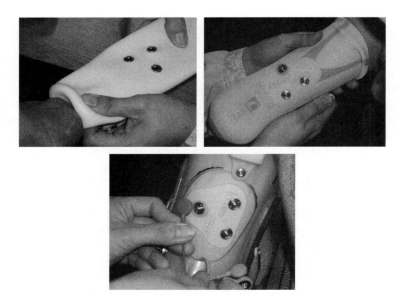

Fig. 15. Roll-on liner with electrodes embedded.

These flexible socket designs distribute force globally, resulting in better overall weight bearing. Flexible interfaces and roll-on suction suspension are incorporated in anatomic contoured sockets. The anatomic contoured socket considers the anatomy and bony structure of the residual limb. Earlier prosthetic devices merely contained the residual limb within the prosthesis. This containment approach necessitated the use of specific harnessing to stabilize the socket. Anatomic contoured sockets can be used in amputations at the styloid, transradial, elbow disarticulation, transhumeral, and shoulder level. Most upper limb–deficient individuals can benefit from these more progressive designs.

The unique anatomy of the styloid and elbow disarticulation amputation level lends itself to an impression technique in which the patients residual limb is submerged in alginate impression material. The resulting mold presents an accurate contour of the patient's residual limb, ensuring a more comfortable prosthetic fit, and is easy to remove owing to the bulbous distal nature of the residual limb. A suction-type design is used to stabilize the residual limb at the contours of the styloids or epicondyles [20].

The transradial anatomic contoured socket contours to the muscles of the residual limb and maintains a suspension that incorporates the benefits of the mediolateral and anterior-posterior contours of the residual limb (Fig. 16). The distinguishing characteristic of this socket design involves intrinsic suspension from contouring of the radioulnar anatomy and musculature, which is a radically different approach than the older practice of extrinsic humeral epicondylar contouring. Intrinsic contouring is superior because it respects the geometric changes throughout the range of elbow motion. In some cases, the authors have modified transradial contoured sockets to a three-quarter type of design to improve air circulation. The contouring of the residual limb also provides for greater stabilization of the radius and ulna within the prosthesis when viewed radiologically (Fig. 17) [21]. Older designs did not address these geometric changes, and as a result amputees had discomfort about the epicondyles.

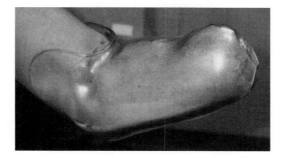

Fig. 16. Transradial anatomic contoured socket.

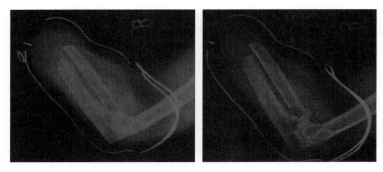

Fig. 17. Radiologic analysis of the TRAC interface without loading (*left*) and with loading (*right*).

The anatomic contoured socket at the transhumeral level is characterized by a reduction in the lateral trim line of the socket and an aggressive modification into the deltopectoral groove anteriorly and a flattened socket just inferior to the spine of scapula (Fig. 18). This type of residual limb contouring provides greater rotation control, enhances range of motion, and reduces the harnessing requirements [22].

At the glenohumeral or associated level of limb deficiency, the microframe shoulder design incorporates socket contours and trim lines that minimize the coverage of the residual limb. This design dissipates heat better and often reduces or eliminates the need to cover the shoulder with any type of rigid plastic. The microframe shoulder design uses anterior-to-posterior compression principles to help maintain suspension of the prosthesis (Fig. 19) [23]. The shoulder level of deficiency exhibits a high rate of rejection from

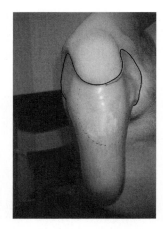

Fig. 18. Transhumeral anatomic contoured socket provides rotation control and enhanced range of motion.

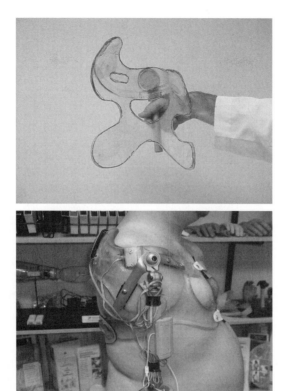

Fig. 19. Microframe provides enhanced suspension and heat dissipation for the glenohumeral and interscapulothoracic deficiency.

variables such as socket discomfort and heat buildup. The microframe design addresses these issues and provides a stable foundation for advanced systems necessary for this highly compromised patient population.

Materials

New prosthetic materials also are improving overall patient comfort. Of particular note is the friction-free donning sock. These socks have been used successfully in lower extremity prosthetics for some time. The socks can be ordered from a manufacturer or can be custom-made based on the patient's residual limb length and size. The socks allow individuals to push into their prosthesis with a minimal amount of friction and pull on the remainder of the socket by use of a lanyard with a contralateral hand or foot (Fig. 20).

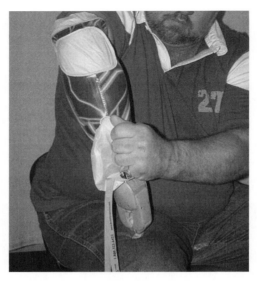

Fig. 20. Use of a donning sock at the transradial level allows for reduced friction during donning and containment of the soft tissues.

Microprocessor technology

Currently, microprocessor technology influences terminal device control; wrist and elbow functions; and other options, such as shoulder joint locking and unlocking, remote on-and-off control, and sensory feedback. Microprocessors illustrate an augmentation to current types of control, not a type of stand-alone control. As a graphic equalizer enhances a complete sound system, the microprocessor delineates filters and enhances input characteristics to produce the desired output optimizing prosthetic function and increasing overall ease of use [24].

Microprocessors provide the ability to modify and enhance control options and input characteristics quickly and easily throughout all phases of upper extremity prosthetic care and product development. Although adjustable microprocessors allow for a faster return to function, they should not take the place of a well-structured rehabilitation plan that focuses on all aspects of upper extremity care from preprosthetic residual limb conditioning to long-term postprosthetic functional goals. Microprocessor use in upper limb prosthetics offers the following benefits [24]:

1. The ability to modify control options and fine-tune input characteristics quickly throughout all stages of prosthetic management without purchasing or exchanging components (eg, Servo/switch control from single site to dual site). This important aspect reduces third-party costs by providing multiple control options in one electronics package.

2. Faster prosthetic fitting and rehabilitation enabling a quicker return to function as encouraged by Malone's guidelines for optimal return to function. Amputees see significant benefits from an early fitting of Servo/switch control with a later transition to single site then to dual site as they move through the preparatory stages of their care.

3. More complex filtering of the electromyogram signal and ease in changing control thresholds and sensitivity of the prosthesis as the user's strength and ability evolves.

4. Real-time input signal analysis providing early detection of residual limb changes.

5. Ability to document and store patient information, allowing for long-term treatment goals to be monitored.

6. Use of complex algorithms to adjust inherently to various situations unknown to the patient, "reducing the mental effort" (Pat Prigge, CP, personal communication, 2000) necessary to function with an electric prosthesis.

7. Incorporation of predefined "behind-the-scenes" programs that monitor and respond to prosthetic functioning. Examples include automatic grasping of the SensorHand (Otto Bock, Minneapolis, MN), autocalibration in the ProControl System (Motion Control, Salt Lake City, UT), and usage monitoring in the Varigrip III processors (Otto Bock, Minneapolis, MN).

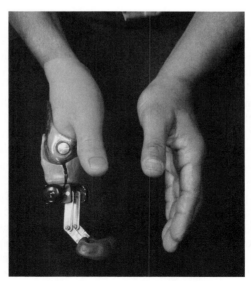

Fig. 21. Advanced Arm Dynamics Electric Partial Hand System. (Courtesy of Advanced Arm Dynamics, Dallas, TX.)

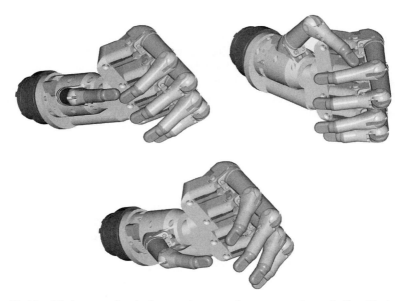

Fig. 22. The iLimb system hand allows various grasping patterns, dramatically widening the scope of the prosthetic terminal device. (Courtesy of Touch EMAS Limited, Edinburgh, UK.)

The aforementioned benefits lead to improved patient functionality and maximization of a patient's rehabilitation potential.

Terminal devices

Two breakthroughs in terminal device technology have had a significant impact on the future of electronic prostheses. The first is the introduction of water/dust resistant components. These new components function better in the real world and have fewer moisture-related problems.

The second major development is that of speed. The Otto Bock Sensor Speed Hand (Otto Bock, Minneapolis, MN) has affected the population with upper limb deficiency dramatically. For the first time, patients feel as if they are no longer waiting for the terminal device to activate. The movement is almost instantaneous with the production of a muscle signal, and that movement shows a higher degree of proportionality to the input signal provided by the patient. The lightning quick and fine-tuned response creates the sensation that the prosthetic limb is truly part of the patient's body.

One focus of renewed interest in the terminal device arena is that of the partial hand level deficiency. Clinically, many patients with an intact thumb and amputation of the remainder of the hand opt to use their sound side instead of a prosthesis, raising concerns that long-term overuse eventually would compromise the intact hand. When using a passive prosthesis at this level, patients consistently voice the wish that prepositioning was unnecessary. The goal at this level is to provide a prosthesis that is completely functional instead of one that requires too much involvement of the sound side. The Advanced Arm Dynamics Electric Partial Hand (Advanced Arm Dynamics, Inc., Dallas, TX) addresses this need and is currently in extended beta site testing (Fig. 21).

Summary

The field of upper extremity prosthetics is a constantly changing arena as researchers and prosthetists strive to bridge the gap between prosthetic reality and upper limb physiology. With the further development of implantable neurologic sensing devices and targeted muscle innervation (discussed elsewhere in this issue), the challenge of limited input to control vast outputs promises to become a historical footnote in the future annals of upper limb prosthetics. Soon multidextrous terminal devices, such as that found in the iLimb system (Touch EMAS, Inc., Edinburgh, UK), will be a clinical reality (Fig. 22). Successful prosthetic care depends on good communication and cooperation among the surgeon, the amputee, the rehabilitation team, and the scientists harnessing the power of technology to solve real-life challenges. If the progress to date is any indication, amputees of the future will find their dreams limited only by their imagination.

Acknowledgments

The authors are grateful to Julie Lake for literary review and editing.

Further readings

Meier RH, Atkins DJ, editors. Functional restoration of adults and children with upper extremity amputation. 2nd edition. New York: Demos Medical Publishing; 2004.
Muzumdar A, editor. Powered upper limb prostheses. Berlin, Germany: Springer; 2004.
Smith DG, Michael JW, Bowker JH, editors. Atlas of amputations and limb deficiencies—surgical, prosthetic and rehabilitation principles. 3rd edition. Rosemont (IL): American Academy of Orthopedic Surgeons; 2004.

References

[1] Atkins DJ, Alley RD. Upper-extremity prosthetics: an emerging specialization in a technologically advanced field. American Occupational Therapy Association 2003. p. CE1–8.
[2] Dillingham TR, Pezzin LE, MacKenzie EJ, et al. Limb deficiency and amputation—epidemiology and recent trends in the US. South Med J 2002;95:875–83.
[3] Brenner CD. Wrist disarticulation and transradial amputation: prosthetic management. In: Smith DG, Michael JW, Bowker JH, editors. Atlas of amputations and limb deficiencies—surgical, prosthetic and rehabilitation principles. 3rd edition. Rosemont (IL): American Academy of Orthopedic Surgeons; 2004. p. 223–30.

[4] Alley RD. Upper limb assessment protocols. Academy Upper Limb Prosthetic Certificate Module; 2001–2003.

[5] Bertals T. Functions of the body harness for upper extremity prostheses. Med Orthop Tech 2001;121:13–7.

[6] Miguelez JM, Conyers D, Zenie J, Lake C. Acute prosthetic upper extremity rehabilitation of blast wound injuries: a 21 month review. In: Conference proceedings of the University of New Brunswick's Myoelectric Controls/Powered Prosthetics Symposium. Fredericton, NB (Canada): University of New Brunswick; 2005. p. 32.

[7] Marquardt E, Neff G. The angulation osteotomy of above-elbow stumps. Clin Orthop 1974; 104:232–8.

[8] Neusel E, Traub M, Blasius K, Marquardt E. Results of humeral stump angulation osteotomy. Arch Orthop Trauma Surg 1997;116:263–5.

[9] Schonhowd TP, Kristensen T, Sivertsen S, Witse E. New technology for the suspension for trans-humeral prostheses—SISA (Subfascial Implant Supported Attachment). In: Conference proceedings of the University of New Brunswick's Myoelectric Controls/Powered Prosthetics Symposium. Fredericton, NB (Canada): University of New Brunswick; 2005. p. 88–92.

[10] Alley RD, Sears HH. Powered upper-limb prosthetics in adults. In: Muzumdar A, editor. Powered upper limb prostheses. New York: Springer; 2004. p. 117–45.

[11] Fletchall S. Returning upper-extremity amputees to work. The O&P Edge 2005;4:28–33.

[12] Jones LE, Davidson JH. Save that arm: a study of problems in the remaining arm of unilateral upper limb amputees. Prosthet Orthot Int 1999;23:55–8.

[13] Sato Y, Kaji M, Oizumi K, et al. Carpal tunnel syndrome involving unaffected limbs of stroke patients. Stroke 1999;30:414–8.

[14] Fraser CM. An evaluation of the use made of cosmetic and functional prostheses by unilateral upper limb amputees. Prosthet Orthot Int 1998;22:216–23.

[15] Davidson J. A comparison of upper limb amputees and patients with upper limb injuries using the disability of the arm shoulder and hand (DASH). In: Conference proceedings of the University of New Brunswick's Myoelectric Controls/Powered Prosthetics Symposium. Fredericton, NB (Canada): University of New Brunswick; 2005. p. 176–82.

[16] Lake C, Miguelez JM. Microprocessors in upper limb prosthetics. Technol Disabil 2003; 15:2.

[17] Lotze M, Grodd W, Birbaumer N, et al. Does use of a myoelectric prosthesis prevent cortical reorganization and phantom limb pain. Nat Neurosci 1999;2:501–2.

[18] Brenner CD. Electric limbs for infants and pre-school children. J Prosthet Orthot 1992;4: 24–30.

[19] Malone JM, et al. Immediate, early and late postsurgical management of upper-limb amputation. J Rehabil Res Dev 1984;21:33–41.

[20] Lake C. Partial hand amputation: prosthetic management. In: Smith DG, Michael JW, Bowker JH, editors. Atlas of amputations and limb deficiencies—surgical, prosthetic and rehabilitation principles. 3rd edition. Rosemont (IL): American Academy of Orthopedic Surgeons; 2004. p. 209–17.

[21] Miguelez JM, Lake C, Conyers D, Zenie J. The transradial anatomically contoured (TRAC) interface: design principles and methodology. J Prosthet Orthot 2003;15:148–56.

[22] Andrew JT. Elbow disarticulation and transhumeral amputation: prosthetic principals. In: Bowker JH, Michael JW, editors. Atlas of limb prosthetics. 2nd edition. St Louis: Mosby Year Book; 1992. p. 255–64.

[23] Miguelez JM, Miguelez MD. The Microframe: the next generation of interface design for glenohumeral disarticulation and associated levels of limb deficiency. J Prosthet Orthot 2003;15:66–71.

[24] Lake C, Miguelez J. Comparative analysis of microprocessors in upper limb prosthetics. J Prosthet Orthot 2003;15:48–63.

PHYSICAL MEDICINE
AND REHABILITATION
CLINICS OF
NORTH AMERICA

ELSEVIER
SAUNDERS

Phys Med Rehabil Clin N Am
17 (2006) 73–89

Comparison Between Custom and Noncustom Spinal Orthoses

Gene P. Bernardoni, CO[a,b,]*, Thomas M. Gavin, CO[c,d]

[a]*Ballert Orthopedic of Chicago, 2434 West Peterson Avenue, Chicago, IL 60659, USA*
[b]*Northwestern University Medical School Prosthetic-Orthotic Center,
Chicago, IL 60611, USA*
[c]*BioConcepts, Inc., 100 Tower Drive, Suite 101, Burr Ridge, IL 60527, USA*
[d]*Musculoskeletal Biomechanics Laboratory, Veterans Administration Hospital,
Hinsdale, IL 60521, USA*

Since initial development in the early 1950s, custom-molded thoracolumbosacral orthoses (TLSOs) have come to be accepted among neurosurgeons and orthopedic surgeons as the best means of controlling spinal motion postoperatively and nonoperatively. Many studies have since been published showing that superior alignment and triplaner motion control can be achieved with custom-molded TLSOs compared with various off-the-shelf (OTS) spinal orthoses.

More recently, numerous companies have begun to market prefabricated (OTS) spinal supports, claiming that they are equivalent to custom-molded TLSOs. After evaluating some of the leading brands of OTS TLSOs with professional staff, other certified orthotists, and numerous orthopedic surgeons and neurosurgeons, the authors conclude, with regard to biomechanical control of motion, patient compliance, and overall cost, that the custom-molded TLSO remains superior to the OTS versions and should remain in most cases the preferred option for postsurgical and trauma patients. If the custom-molded high-profile or low-profile (which some OTS manufacturers call a lumbosacral orthosis [LSO]) TLSO is considered overbracing in light of improved instrumentation, and less motion control is needed, many less expensive options exist, including the standard lumbosacral corset. This article explains the reasoning behind the authors' conclusions. The authors compared OTS spinal supports with the custom-molded TLSO in five basic areas: biomechanics, fit, compliance, cost, and liability.

---

* Corresponding author. Ballert Orthopedic of Chicago, 2434 West Peterson Avenue, Chicago, IL 60659, USA.
E-mail address: info@ballert-op.com (G.P. Bernardoni).

1047-9651/06/$ - see front matter © 2006 Elsevier Inc. All rights reserved.
doi:10.1016/j.pmr.2005.10.005   *pmr.theclinics.com*

Biomechanical considerations

Generally, custom orthoses fit the patient more intimately than OTS ortho-ses by virtue of the fact that they are molded to each patient's body. In contrast to the completely circumferential custom-molded TLSO, the OTS spinal sup-port usually consists of a shallow anterior and posterior panel connected with adjustment straps or thin plastic tongues or an anterior opening similar to a lumbosacral corset. Although manufacturers may claim biomechanical equivalence with custom appliances, the authors have found significant defi-ciencies in biomechanical effectiveness among OTS spinal supports. Some OTS appliances may approach the custom-molded TLSO with regard to in-tracavitary pressure and kinesthetic withdrawal [1], but they are not equiva-lent in controlling triplanar motion; OTS appliances focus on flexion and extension only. Even so, in many cases, because of the soft shell or anterior opening, the flexion/extension of OTS appliances is compromised compared with custom orthoses. In virtually all cases, OTS orthoses do not or very poorly control lateral flexion and rotation, whereas custom orthoses are able to control these motions quite well. Why OTS orthoses fail to achieve the tripla-nar motion control of custom-molded TLSOs is discussed subsequently.

Immobilization

Sagittal plane motion

Sagittal plane motion is controlled by the anterior and posterior panels of the orthosis working together. The height of the panels (vertical lever arm length), the stiffness of the material from which the orthosis is made, and the integrity of the panel all combine to inhibit motion. The anterior panel inhibits spinal flexion, and the posterior panel inhibits spinal extension. One can see that a high anterior panel would prevent anterior flexion of the lum-bar or thoracic spine, whereas a high posterior panel would prevent poste-rior extension of the thoracic or lumbar spine. In both cases, the opposite panel or a simple narrow strap sets up a three-point pressure system (Fig. 1).

Many OTS spinal orthoses have a posterior shell that is higher than the anterior shell, encouraging a flexion moment (Fig. 2). This low anterior trimline is contraindicated in most nonoperative or postsurgical conditions. A superior anterior trimline at or slightly below the superior end of a poste-rior fusion with instrumentation is not only ineffective in prohibiting flexion at the most vulnerable point of the fusion, but it also acts as a fulcrum that could increase the flexion force and lead to failure, as shown in Fig. 2. Most surgeons agree that a posterior implant is most vulnerable by uncontrolled anterior flexion [2]. Maintaining a neutral spinal alignment and prohibiting anterior flexion protect the implant. In many cases, a longer anterior shell with a shorter posterior shell is indicated to encourage an extension moment (see Fig. 1). Only in disease conditions such as spondylolisthesis or in con-ditions in which it is beneficial to unload the posterior column, such as

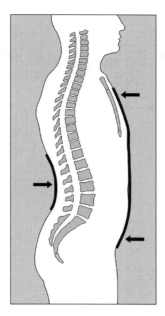

Fig. 1. Three-point pressure system. (Courtesy of Ballert Orthopedic; with permission.)

spinal arthritis or nerve root entrapment, is it indicated to encourage a flexion moment. Most OTS spinal supports do not address the fact that different conditions require different sagittal plane alignments.

Coronal plane motion

The lateral panels of an orthosis control coronal plane motion. These panels act in the same way as the anterior and posterior panels described earlier. The longer or higher the panel, the better motion can be controlled. Lateral flexion is more limited by the anatomy (locked facet joints with normal lumbar lordosis) than is anterior flexion. The lateral panels of an Aspen LSO (Aspen Medical Products, Inc., Irvine, California) also are lower (the overlapping outer panel is the effective lateral height, not the soft polyethylene inner panel and foam liner [see Fig. 2]) than on a lumbosacral corset or a low-profile TLSO, and this deficiency allows for greater lateral flexion, which may be a detriment to patient outcomes. OTS spinal supports that use only straps or thin polyethylene tongues laterally also cannot control lateral flexion as well as the firm lateral panels of a custom-molded TLSO (Fig. 3). This is a serious flaw in the treatment of spondylolisthesis because it has been shown that this motion was the most detrimental [3].

Transverse plane motion

The most effective means of controlling rotation is a high-profile trimline with subclavicular extensions that act with the contralateral anterior

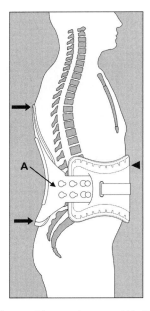

Fig. 2. Aspen low-profile appliance with extender strap (A). (Courtesy of Ballert Orthopedic; with permission.)

superior iliac spine (ASIS) (Fig. 4). The high trimline is necessary to control motion in the thoracic and lumbar spine from T6 to L4. Rotation in the L5-S1 area is best controlled with a low-profile TLSO with hip spica. In a low-profile TLSO, it is necessary to encompass the ribs and have a good lock on the

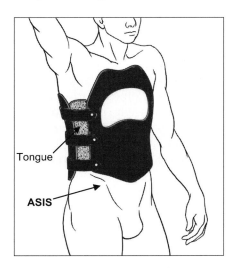

Fig. 3. VertAlign (Bremer Group Co., Jacksonville, FL) with polyethylene tongue. (Courtesy of Ballert Orthopedic; with permission.)

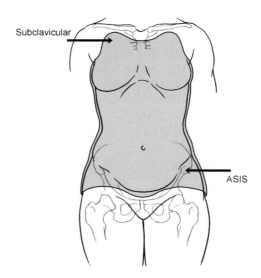

Fig. 4. Derotation principle. Custom-molded TLSO with contact at ASIS and subclavicular area. (Courtesy of Ballert Orthopedic; with permission.)

pelvis and ASIS to control rotation (see Fig. 4). For this reason, an LSO below the ribs does not control rotation as well as a custom-molded TLSO that encompasses the ribs because the attempted rotation is stopped by the contralateral ASIS. Many OTS TLSOs do not cover the ASIS (see Fig. 3). To inhibit rotation, an orthosis must make contact with ribs and ASIS. In the posterior spinal fusion with or without instrumentation in the high lumbar and thoracic regions, rotation is the second most detrimental force that can lead to failure. Subclavicular trimlines are needed in Harrington rod–like instrumentations to stop rotation that could allow the superior hooks to dislodge. The subclavicular extension also is a good kinesthetic reminder to limit anterior reach or shoulder flexion. The authors have seen patients who get up at night, forget to put on the orthosis, and open the refrigerator to get a glass of milk. The patient leans forward, flexes the shoulder, and extends the elbow, so they now have a significant flexion moment across the surgical site. This is amplified by the arm extended with a gallon of milk, causing failure. Custom-molded TLSOs are designed to prevent this kind of failure, whereas OTS appliances are lacking in this area.

With the Aspen high-profile TLSO, the thoracic section is connected to the LSO pelvic section by means of the round rods, which cannot control rotation because the rods twist, superimposing one over the other, allowing rotation at the junction of the two sections. Many surgeons believe that rotational control is not as crucial in newer implant systems that use screws at each vertebral level, although gross twisting motions with long lever arms (rotation) can put large torque loads on the screws at the level of maximum spinal rotational motion (usually at the T12-L1 junction). On the rare occasions when new constructs fail, they do so as a result of combined flexion and rotation.

The series of photographs in Fig. 5 graphically illustrates the superior ability of custom TLSOs over OTS braces when it comes to controlling spinal rotation. In Fig. 5A, the unbraced subject lifts the shoulder off the examination table (horizontal flexion) while keeping the spine, pelvis, and posterior ribs flat on the table. In each case, this is done by the examiner pushing down on both

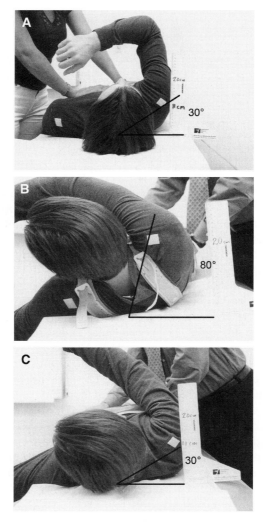

Fig. 5. (*A*) An unbraced subject shows pure shoulder motion (30°). (*B*) Wearing the Aspen brace, the subject adds spinal rotation of roughly 50°. (*C*) Wearing the custom-molded TLSO, the subject's spinal motion is restricted to 0°. Only horizontal flexion of the shoulder is visible. (Courtesy of Ballert Orthopedic; with permission.)

ASIS to keep the pelvis flat on the examination table. In Fig. 5B, the subject next attempts to rotate maximally off the examination table while wearing an Aspen TLSO with the pelvis held flat on the examination table. In Fig. 5C, the subject attempts to rotate maximally with a custom-molded TLSO with the pelvis held flat on the table. Although pure shoulder motion (30°) is allowed under all scenarios, shoulder and spinal rotation measuring roughly 80° is allowed with the Aspen TLSO (ie, 50° of spinal rotation).

Angulation

Kinematics

Although much attention has been given to the ability of spinal orthoses to reduce planar motion, more current thinking has clinicians considering the ability of orthoses to change planar alignment, specific to injury or instability.

Nonoperative fractures

It may be derived from the literature that orthoses for the nonoperative management of spinal fractures must be able to hyperextend the injury site. They should yield a radiographically measurable increase in height of the front of the spine at the fracture site. This increase in height closes facet joints posteriorly and tenses the anterior longitudinal ligament and anterior annulus, resisting progression of the deformity, while immobilizing the injured site in all three planes. The orientation of these biologic components being compressed posteriorly and tensed anteriorly would be the *best* method of immobilizing the nonoperative spinal fracture. Also, to manage a burst fracture effectively [4], for example, the orthosis may need 65° of lumbar hyperlordosis to (1) address the gibbus, (2) restore vertebral height, and (3) open the vertebral foramen. No OTS appliance accounts for this aggressive sagittal positioning. Containment of the torso in a plastic tube (such as is afforded by all OTS appliances) does not guarantee immobilization or resistance to injury progression.

Stenosis

The inverse is true for patients with stenosis, but for different reasons. The posterior aspect of the spine requires tension, whereas the anterior aspect requires compression. Although this opens facet joints and transfers loading on the disk, this pathology is neurocompressive, and the hyperflexion is necessary to decompress neural elements that are trapped by anatomic artifacts. This is not a "classic" instability and must be hyperangulated into flexion. For fractures and stenosis/spondylolisthesis, it is important to hyperangulate the spine to the maximum potential of each patient. The authors question the ability of OTS spinal orthoses to achieve optimal angulation.

Spondylolysis and Spondylolisthesis

It is accepted protocol to treat spondylolysis and grades I and II spondylo-listhesis with an orthosis [5–8]. Originally, three biomechanical factors were thought to affect bony union and reduce pain: abdominal intracavitary pressure, posterior pelvic tilt, and reduction or lordosis. Williams [9] showed that reduction in lordosis (an extension stop in sagittal plane) and inducing posterior pelvic tilt were necessary to treat these conditions effectively (Fig. 6). Williams [9] also showed that allowing flexion was beneficial. He stated that intra-abdominal pressure may be harmful in that it weakens the abdominal musculature needed to maintain the posterior pelvic tilt after the orthosis was removed. Reduced lordosis and posterior pelvic tilt again were proven to be effective by Hall et al [10] in a study with the Boston overlap brace

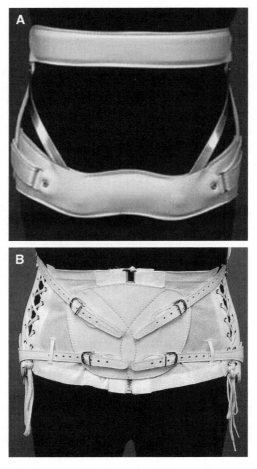

Fig. 6. Williams orthosis. Posterior (*A*) and anterior (*B*) views. (Courtesy of Boston Brace; with permission.)

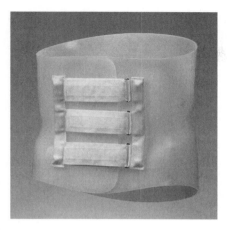

Fig. 7. Boston overlap brace. (Courtesy of Truform OTC; with permission.)

(Boston Brace International, Inc., Avon, Massachusetts) (Fig. 7) and by others [11–14]. In contrast to the OTS supports mentioned in this article and many other OTS supports, the researchers in the Boston study recognized that there are variations in the amount of lordosis from individual to individual and manufactured three different lordotic curve patterns. To custom mold a posterior shell in an antilordotic angle, the patient must be cast either supine or seated with the knees higher than the hips. The posterior shell must extend from 24 mm inferior to the inferior angle of the scapula to the gluteal crease. There must be lateral indentations superior to the iliac crest and inferior to the inferior costal margin (at the natural waist) to ensure that the orthosis does not migrate superiorly when the patient sits. The anterior shell must be shorter to allow flexion, and there should be a firm posterior force on the ASIS to affect posterior pelvic tilt [3]. None of the OTS supports mentioned in this article conform to the rigorous angulation standards needed for effective treatment of these conditions. The posterior shells are not long enough (superiorly or inferiorly) to hold the patient maximally in an antilordotic posture. The abbreviated wire frame posterior piece of the Aspen support not only is not long enough, but also is centrally located in such a way as to allow a patient to roll laterally into extension. None of the OTS supports have deep lateral indentations to prevent migration of the orthosis, and consequently they migrate superiorly when the patient sits and in general do not maintain their position of the body.

Postoperative/postfusion

The task of a surgical implant is to immobilize a segment while a bone graft grows into a solid fusion mass, obliterating motion, over time, at that segment. The vulnerability of any implant is that implants are always significantly stiffer than the bone to which they are attached. A postoperative orthosis that does not perfectly match the postoperative geometry of the spine may be creating artifact forces that may influence loosening of an implant. This is especially true for elderly patients, who already may have compromised bone mineral density, increasing the differences between the bone and implant stiffnesses [15]. Most OTS orthoses are made in fixed geometries that are not hyperextended or hyperflexed and are not able to match a postoperative fusion construct alignment reliably.

Fit considerations

Most manufacturers of OTS TLSOs offer a choice of only several sizes. They usually do not consider differences in lordosis and rarely consider gender anatomic differences or obese patients (Fig. 8). People of different ethnic origins exhibit body differences, such as long or short waistedness. Some clinicians attempt to compensate for the restrictive choice of sizes by using shallow concave anterior and posterior shells and a series of straps or straps and thin polyethylene tongues to join them (see Fig. 3). Others use an anterior opening (eg, lumbosacral corset) with extender strap to accommodate different circumferences (see Fig. 2).

In terms of fit, there are several drawbacks to this approach. First, a TLSO with shallow concave shells is ineffective in controlling the movement in overweight and obese patients, a group estimated to constitute 70% of the adult US population. OTS spinal supports do not include a good pouch for pendulous abdomens, whereas a custom-molded orthosis can accommodate them easily. The failure to accommodate the abdomen

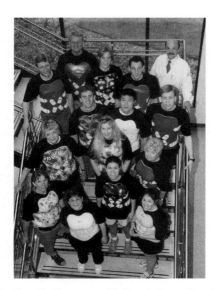

Fig. 8. One size fits all? (Courtesy of Ballert Orthopedic; with permission.)

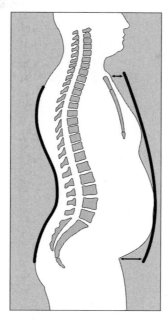

Fig. 9. Flat anterior shell does not fit abdomen. (Courtesy of Ballert Orthopedic; with permission.)

prevents contact at the sternum and symphysis pubis, which compromises control of motion, especially flexion/extension (Fig. 9). The effective vertical lever arm length measures from the superior-most contact point to the inferior-most contact point. An abdominal "spare tire" acts as a ball bearing to a flat anterior panel and does not allow the orthosis to make contact on the sternum or symphysis pubis. A custom-formed pouch also allows compression and intracavitary pressure without allowing the excess tissue to slip under the anterior inferior edge of the TLSO. In a custom-molded TLSO, such a pouch also helps to keep the orthosis from migrating superiorly because the iliac crest pads or indentations do not work as well by themselves in an obese individual. In the OTS spinal support, by contrast, the absence of the pendulous abdomen pouch forces excess tissue to push under the inferior edge of the anterior shell (Fig. 10). This excess tissue may well cause the orthosis to migrate superiorly, while forfeiting the biomechanical principle of elevating intracavitary pressure to provide axial unloading.

In the custom-molded TLSO, the authors normally create a deep indentation over the iliac crest and continuing medial to the ASIS. This is something that is missing in OTS spinal supports (Fig. 11). Achieved by modifying a deep groove in the positive model of the patient or adding a foam crest pad, such an indentation is extremely important in preventing the migration of the orthosis superiorly and preventing rotation of the

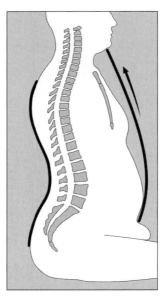

Fig. 10. Flat anterior shell causes excess abdominal tissue to escape under shell. (Courtesy of Ballert Orthopedic; with permission.)

orthosis on the body [3]. In custom TLSOs, the authors modify this waist groove deeply and may add foam crest pads to ensure a good lock on the pelvis and increase end-point control. Effective end-point control helps to increase the load-carrying capacity of the spine. If these waist grooves are not deep enough or the patient wears the orthosis too loose, the whole

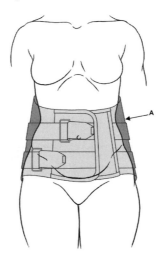

Fig. 11. The Cybertec (Bio Cypernetics International, LaVerne, CA) appliance does not conform to the patient's waist (A). (Courtesy of Ballert Orthopedic; with permission.)

orthosis migrates or rotates. Configuration and depth of the waist modification are determined by the anatomy of the patient and the firmness of the patient's tissue; this can be ascertained only by actually seeing, measuring, and casting the patient. Because this assessment cannot be done for OTS spinal supports, their waist grooves are shallow or do not exist at all, allowing these supports to migrate when the patient sits or to rotate on the patient. In either case, the orthosis is no longer in the desired position to control motion at the specified vertebral level.

OTS spinal orthoses are not to be ruled out in all clinical situations. For some nonsurgical conditions (eg, anterior compression fractures), in which hyperextension of the patient is desirable, a high-profile spinal orthosis, such as Jewett-like hyperextension braces or the cruciform anterior sternal hyperextension orthosis (CASH), work quite well. Both of these are more economical than the new crop of OTS TLSOs. Orthoses that provide kinesthetic withdrawal or intracavitary pressure for axial unloading, such as lumbosacral corsets, Warm 'N Form, Aspen LSO, and Cybertech LSO, also are appropriate within their indicated limitations. The Aspen and Cybertec are substantially more expensive than the others, however, without providing a greater degree of control. The Cybertec closure system is superior to others in providing an easy tightening mechanism for individuals who have compromised upper extremity strength.

Although the manufacturers of OTS spinal supports claim that they are biomechanically equivalent to custom-molded TLSOs, this is usually true only with regard to kinesthetic withdrawal and intracavitary pressure. Although they may control motion in the sagittal plane, they cannot control motion in all planes as well as the custom orthoses (especially lacking in motion control in the coronal and transverse planes). Their failure to address adequately anatomic gender differences, body type differences, the numerous overweight and obese patients, and kyphotic and lordotic differences among patients compromises their ability to control motion or even spinal alignment.

Compliance

It is self-evident that an orthosis cannot do the therapeutic job it is designed to perform unless the patient wears it. Patients tend to avoid wearing their braces for one of three reasons: (1) The brace is uncomfortable to wear; (2) it causes embarrassment; or (3) the patient does not understand how to wear the brace properly.

Comfort factor

Because they are custom formed to the patient's body, custom-molded TLSOs are usually more comfortable to wear than are OTS orthoses. The custom TLSO restricts motion, which is what it is designed to do. It is necessary to explain this to the patient. The motion restriction may be something the patient does not like at first, but they usually adjust to it in a short time. Although patients sometimes complain that the plastic is hot, it is not hotter than OTS orthoses that use thin polyethylene and 3/8-inch foam liner (Aspen LSO). Cybertec is perforated in an attempt to allow heat dissipation. The authors address this in custom-molded TLSOs by drilling holes to dissipate the heat. From the standpoint of heat, lumbosacral corset or open-frame orthoses are coolest. Even if an OTS brace is marginally more comfortable, the physician must consider carefully the tradeoff between comfort and effective restriction of motion.

Embarrassment factor

Most OTS orthoses are bulkier than custom orthoses and do not lend themselves to being worn under clothes. A TLSO with a liner can and should be worn under clothes. Although it does not happen often, the authors have been able to accommodate patients without compromising function of the orthosis. The authors once made a custom-molded hyperextension TLSO to be worn under a sleeveless gown (Fig. 12). With the exception of tight-fitting clothes such as jeans, most individuals have clothes that fit over custom orthoses. The authors instruct patients to wear the TLSO with only a stockinet (provided with all TLSOs), T-shirt, or tube underneath and to put their clothes (including panties or shorts) over the TLSO.

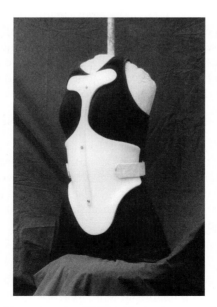

Fig. 12. Custom-molded hyperextension TLSO with aluminum anterior bar inside plastic for rigidity. (Courtesy of Ballert Orthopedic; with permission.)

Donning/doffing factor

Because they depend so much on a multiplicity of straps, OTS orthoses are much more complex for the patient to put on and adjust than are custom-made orthoses. In an effort to compensate for the limited number of sizes, manufacturers of OTS orthoses have added a dizzying series of straps and buckles intended to permit a finer-tuned fit. The Aspen TLSO has seven straps to attach and adjust. In the case of the Aspen TLSO or LSO, the straps make it difficult to learn to apply properly, even for trained orthotists. This complexity means that patients often are unable to adjust their orthoses for maximum benefit and may give up wearing them entirely out of frustration with all the straps that need adjusting. Although all orthoses require some patient training, the authors have tried to eliminate patient guesswork in application by using labeling, straightforward instructions, and the characteristics of the orthosis itself so that the orthosis can be applied time after time with proper orientation and the same degree of compression.

Cost

In light of the biomechanical and compliance deficiencies, it is surprising to learn that OTS spinal supports *cost more* than custom-molded TLSOs. The cost to the hospital or to the patient of an OTS appliance is frequently higher than a custom orthosis. In the case of the Aspen TLSOs, the cost to the hospital is frequently $300 to $400 more than the custom TLSO, including the cost of follow-up visits. More follow-up visits are required with an OTS appliance. When an Aspen is used in place of a lumbosacral corset or a Warn 'N Form, the former can cost $500 to $600 more. When the hospital cannot pass along the cost of the item to the patient's insurance, as in a diagosis-related group or per diem stay, the cost falls directly to the hospital's bottom line.

When these OTS supports are used in nonoperative treatment of spinal conditions, they fail to reduce motion sufficiently, resulting in pain for the patient. This frequently requires the fitting of a custom TLSO to get satisfactory results. In these cases, the patient or his or her insurance must pay for two orthoses. Although clinicians should not consider cost at the expense of clinical outcome, they would be remiss to pay dearly for poor or inferior clinical outcomes.

Liability

In the attempt to shore up decreasing reimbursement rates, physicians sometimes are lured into fitting noncustom spinal supports. Many times they are fitted by an untrained staff person, not the physician himself or herself. This situation exposes the physician to additional liability. Having the knowledge that a particular orthosis is not as effective as another in controlling motion and using the inferior orthosis may expose one to liability in the event of the failure of a fusion, further progression of an injury, or improper alignment causing neurologic impairment. Usually a certified orthotist is called into court cases as an expert witness, and his or her testimony is typically given greater weight over other witnesses who do not have a degree or license in orthotics. In Chicago, the Director of the Orthotic Program at Northwestern University Prosthetic and Orthotic School is often called as an expert witness.

A second possible area of vulnerability in any court hearing is the use of a noncertified or nonlicensed orthotist in the fitting of an orthosis. There are specific rules dictated by the American Board for Certification and the Illinois Orthotic and Prosthetic Board as to the various types of supervision required when allowing medical personnel other than a certified orthotist to measure for and fit an orthosis. Salespeople for various manufacturers of orthotic devices usually are not certified or licensed orthotists and have no training whatsoever other than sales training.

Summary

Although economically priced OTS orthoses can and should be used under certain prescribed conditions to satisfy carefully described treatment objectives, they cannot control motion as well as custom-molded TLSOs. Patients should not pay for expensive products that cannot help to ensure the best possible clinical outcome. The custom-molded TLSO provides superior fit and support relative to its OTS relative and induces better compliance among its wearers because of its simplicity. It is also the most cost-effective option.

Acknowledgments

For reading early drafts and making suggestions that resulted in an improved article, the authors are grateful to Aruna Ganju, MD, Department of Neurosurgery, Northwestern Memorial Hospital; Fred Geisler, MD, founder of the Illinois Neurological Spine Center at Rush-Copley Medical Center; Purnendu Gupta, MD, Department of Orthopedics, The University of Chicago Hospitals; Bryan Malas, CO, Director of the orthotics and prosthetics program at Northwestern University; Steven M. Mardjetko, MD, FAAP, Illinois Bone and Joint; and Paul R. Meyer, MD, Professor of Orthopedic Surgery, Northwestern University.

References

[1] Cholewicki J, Juhuru K, Radebold A, et al. Lumbar spine stability can be augmented with an abdominal belt and/or increased intra-abdominal pressure. Eur Spine J 1999;8:388–95.

[2] Lorenz M, Patwardhan A, Zindrick M. Instability and mechanics of implants and braces for thoracic and lumbar fractures. In: Errico T, editor. Spinal trauma. Philadelphia: Lippincott; 1990. p. 271–80.

[3] Smith KM. A preliminary report on a new design of spinal orthosis for spondylotic patients: review of the literature and initiation for future study of a new design. J Prosthet Orthot 1998; 10:45.

[4] Knight RQ, Stornelli DP, Chan DPK, et al. Comparison of operative versus nonoperative treatment of lumbar burst fractures. Clin Orthop 1993;293:112–21.

[5] Teitz CC, Hu SS, Arendt EA. The female athlete: evaluation and treatment of sports-related problems. J Am Acad Orthop Surg 1997;5:87–96.

[6] Wiltse LL, Newman PH, Macnab I. Classification of spondylolysis and spondylolisthesis. Clin Orthop 1976;117:23–9.

[7] Soren A, Waugh TR. Spondylolisthesis and related disorders: a correlative study of 105 patients. Clin Orthop 1985;193:171–7.

[8] Micheli LJ, Hall JE, Miller ME. Use of modified Boston brace for back injuries in athletes. Am J Sports Med 1980;8:351–9.

[9] Williams PC. The conservative management of lesions of the lumbosacral spine. Instr Course Lect 1953;10:90–102.

[10] Hall JE, Miller ME, Cassella MC, et al. Manual for the Boston Brace Workshop. Boston: Department of Orthopedics, Children's Hospital; 1976.

[11] Steiner ME, Micheli LJ. Treatment of symptomatic spondylolysis and spondylolisthesis with the modified Boston brace. Spine 1985;10:937–43.

[12] Bell DF, Ehrlich MG, Zaleske DJ. Brace treatment of symptomatic spondylolisthesis: retrospective comparison and three-year follow-up of two conservative treatment programs. Arch Phys Med Rehabil 1989;70:594–8.

[13] Pizzutillo PD, Hummer CD III. Nonoperative treatment for painful adolescent spondylolysis and spondylolisthesis. J Pediatr Orthop 1989;9:538–40.

[14] d'Hemecourt PA. Spondylolysis: returning the athlete to sports participation with brace treatment. Orthopedics 2002;25:653–7.

[15] Harrington PR. Treatment of scoliosis, correction and internal fixation by spine instrumentation. J Bone Joint Surg Am 1962;44:591–610.

ELSEVIER
SAUNDERS

Phys Med Rehabil Clin N Am
17 (2006) 91–113

PHYSICAL MEDICINE
AND REHABILITATION
CLINICS OF
NORTH AMERICA

Microprocessor Prosthetic Knees

Dale Berry, CP, FAAOP

*Clinical Operations, Hanger Orthopedic Group, 820 North Lilac Drive,
Suite 110, Golden Valley, MN 55422, USA*

During the 1970s, research in the field of computerized knee joints began in the university environment. In the late 1980s and early 1990s, various prosthetic companies began working on the first commercial microprocessor controlled knee joints. The initial computerized designs focused on having the microprocessor control and influence the swing phase of gait—the time of gait that begins when the foot leaves the floor as the knee is flexing and ends when that same foot contacts the ground again at heel-strike. These initial systems received mixed acceptance within the health care and amputee community because although the knees increased walking speed and improved the ability to change walking speeds quickly, the knees did not provide any improvement over existing technology with regard to stability and security during stance phase of gait—the time when the prosthetic foot is in contact with the ground from heel-strike to toe-off.

In the late 1990s, new models of microprocessor knees were introduced to the market that provided swing phase control with the addition of stance phase control [1,2]. This improvement dramatically increased the acceptance and application of this technology as it addressed the stability and functional needs of transfemoral amputees with regard to performing activities of daily living (Table 1) [3,4].

The primary benefits of the microprocessor swing and stance control knee mechanism is to improve the overall balance of the wearer and provide a higher degree of confidence and reliance with the prosthetic knee [5–7]. The wearer has confidence to walk down ramps and stairs step over step, traverse uneven terrain, and walk with variable cadence and has the freedom to pursue a normal and active lifestyle without having to concentrate on each and every step with the prosthesis to perform activities of daily living.

E-mail address: Dale.Berry@Hanger.com

1047-9651/06/$ - see front matter © 2006 Elsevier Inc. All rights reserved.
doi:10.1016/j.pmr.2005.10.006

Table 1
Activities of daily living

Activity of daily living	Microprocessor knee design feature
Walk with variable cadence (change walking speeds)	The microprocessor monitors and assesses the ambulatory moments of the prosthesis at a rate of 50–1000 times/s. The knee senses changes in gait speed in real time and makes immediate and necessary adjustments to the flexion and extension resistance to ensure optimal stability and knee movement regardless of gait speed. The knee instantaneously self-adjusts to enable secure and natural gait patterns from a very slow gait to high-speed walking and running
Walk long distances	Gait with a microprocessor knee is more natural, symmetric, and energy efficient owing to the knee continuously monitoring and adjusting to gait speed, ground conditions, and stability requirements. The microprocessor readjusts the flexion resistance during stance phase to nearly effortless knee bending to initiate pre swing in less than 1/10 of a second to provide a smooth natural knee motion during swing phase. Reduced energy consumption prolongs the time it takes the muscles to fatigue
Walk on uneven terrain (gravel, grass, curbs)	The microprocessor continually monitors ambulatory moments of the prosthesis and immediately identifies and reacts to unnatural or inappropriate knee and ankle movements, strain, or stress. Within 1/10 of a second after identifying an unnatural movement or strain, the knee is adjusted to maximum stance resistance to ensure the knee is providing optimal stability for the situation
Descend stairs	The stance flexion-yielding rate can decelerate the prosthesis while descending stairs. The microprocessor stance control and stumble recovery settings or specific yield settings programmed for stairs descent provide optimal resistance for decelerating knee flexion to enable step-over-step descending of stairs
Descend ramps	Advanced stumble recovery and ramp descent detection sensors, combined with the stance flexion design, enable the wearer to initiate heel strike during the gait cycle with the knee in a natural and flexed position. This feature with "flexion dampening" mimics the normal gait cycle of the anatomic knee even during ramp descent
Carry or lift items (ie, books, infant, groceries)	Independent software-modulated control of swing phase flexion resistance, adjusted at rates from 50–1000 times/s, means that the artificial limb identifies additional loads and the change in the overall center of gravity created by the additional load and provides the appropriate and optimal stability
Walk in public areas or crowds	With the computer continually assessing gait and walking conditions, the person does not need to control continuously and consciously all movements of the knee with muscular control. This contributes to a significant reduction in overall energy consumption regardless of ground conditions or gait speed

Table 1 (*continued*)

Activity of daily living	Microprocessor knee design feature
Getting in and out of a car	The microprocessor knee allows the person to bear weight on the prosthesis while in a flexed position. This significantly reduces strain and stress on the lower back and sound limb. It also reduces the dependence on the upper limbs to support the body while entering or exiting a car
Bending and sitting	The microprocessor knee allows the person to bear weight on the prosthesis while in a flexed position. This resistance greatly reduces the stress and strain on the sound limb and lower back. The wearer can use both lower limbs to achieve a seated position
Stationary standing	The microprocessor is designed to allow the individual to bear weight on the prosthesis while in a flexed position that mimics the knee position of a sound limb in a stationary or standing position. This enables the wearer to maintain normal hip and low back skeletal and muscular posture

How microprocessor knees work

In a sound limb during swing phase, the muscles of the thigh control the angular motion at the knee joint in flexion and extension. During normal human locomotion, the muscles of the thigh react with different intensities of contraction when changes in gait speed occur. During stance phase, the muscles of the lower limb contract to prevent the knee from collapsing and to influence the lower limb joints to maintain forward momentum of the body. At a higher gait speed, the muscles contract with greater intensity to move the limb at a faster rate. At a lower gait speed, a less intense contraction is needed to move the limb at a lower speed.

With a prosthetic knee joint, the ability to control the flexion/extension speed and resistance of the knee is achieved with a fluid control system; pneumatic or hydraulic valves provide resistance to fluid flow and control the flexion and extension speed at the knee. Nonmicroprocessor knees are designed with valves that require a manual adjustment and are set by the prosthetist during the fitting process of the prosthesis. The challenge presented with this style of mechanical knee mechanism is that the knee cannot assess the person's gait pattern to make immediate or dramatic adjustments that may be necessary to accommodate changes in walking speed and environmental obstacles during normal locomotion.

Microprocessor knees use the same fundamental hydraulic and pneumatic fluid control systems that are integrated with nonmicroprocessor knees. Instead of manually adjusted settings within the knee to accommodate a wide variety of activities of daily living, the microprocessor knee uses a series of sensors to monitor the knee position and function and performs immediate and necessary flexion and extension resistance adjustments to ensure the knee is maintained in the optimal setting for the wearer [8].

Microprocessor knees use sensors and electronic monitoring systems to analyze the patient's gait pattern continuously to control the resistance to knee flexion at different gait speeds [9]. Proper foot clearance and timing are ensured during swing phase. If the knee flexion speed is low, the sensors input the readings into the microprocessor. The microprocessor calculates the optimal settings and automatically adjusts the valve controls in the knee to the appropriate resistance. This technology requires an energy source to power the sensors, microprocessor, and Servo motors that adjust the valves. Lithium ion battery technology provides a small reliable power source that requires recharging on a regular basis. Although some styles of microprocessor knees have a battery that can last 15 days between recharging, it is recommended that the wearer habitually charge the knee once a day to ensure the knee is always fully charged at the beginning of a day.

The onboard computer of the microprocessor knee collects data from two separate sensors within the prosthesis at a rate of 50 to 1000 times/s. The first set of sensors monitors the knee angle position, by taking repetitive readings of the knee flexion angle: The computer can determine if the knee is flexing or extending, or if the readings are constant, the computer determines if the knee is stationary. The second set of force sensors measures the amount of rotational stress or force applied below the knee during gait. During heel-strike, a plantar-flexion moment is applied to the foot, which creates an anterior rotational force, and conversely, toe-off creates a dorsiflexion moment that generates a posterior rotation force (Fig. 1).

The data collected from the knee angle sensor and the force sensors are processed and analyzed by the microprocessor continuous gait assessment function (also referred to as *gait assessment algorithms*). This function

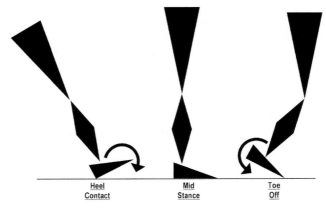

Fig. 1. Ankle and knee rotational forces. At heel-strike, the foot experiences an anterior rotation force creating a plantar flexion influence. At toe-off, the foot experiences a posterior rotational moment creating a dorsiflexion influence. (Courtesy of Hanger Orthopedic Group, Inc., Bethesda, MD.)

examines the data and determines if the knee angle position and forces applied about the knee or foot are within appropriate parameters for normal human gait. Based on the knee position and applied forces, the microprocessor can identify whether the wearer is in swing phase or stance phase. The system also can identify changes in gait speed, determine if the wearer is on stairs, ramps, or uneven terrain; is stationary; or is taking an unnatural step and is about to fall or stumble. From the data collected by the sensors and the analysis of the information by the continuous gait assessment function, the microprocessor knee is able to adjust the knee function within 1/100 of a second to increase or decrease the knee resistance to ensure the knee is in the optimal stability and functional setting for the wearer at all times.

The angle of knee flexion is regulated to mimic the knee more closely during normal gait at varying walking speeds. This ability to change the fluid resistance automatically during gait enables the individual to mimic the normal human function of increased or decreased muscle contraction intensity. Gait is more natural.

With the microprocessor knee, the wearer can maintain active control of the knee during stance phase. Microprocessor controlled knee joints have various control programs and sensors that continuously detect which part of the gait cycle the wearer is in and predicts when stance phase will be initiated. The computer system uses force sensors to assess the gait patterns at a rate of 50 to 1000 times/s and can make instantaneous adjustments to the knee action and resistance to flexion.

When stance phase is initiated, the microprocessor ensures that resistance to knee flexion is high so that the knee does not collapse during stance phase. Security is enhanced by decreasing the risk of falling. Also, the need for physiologically unsound compensatory movements during walking is reduced.

A microprocessor-controlled knee joint can detect movements that are not part of the normal gait pattern. It can activate a higher resistance to flexion, helping to prevent a fall and potential injury. In this way, the microprocessor-controlled knee joint can provide greater security and stability for the individuals on many different types of terrain and with activities of daily living.

What microprocessor knees do

The fundamental design of the microprocessor knee is to enable a transfemoral amputee the ability to accomplish activities of normal daily living with security and safety, while reducing the degree of stress to the sound limb and other joints related to ambulation [10]. The primary focus is to provide a safe and functional prosthetic device to react and respond to the patient's gait pattern in swing and stance phase of human gait (Fig. 2).

The increase in energy requirements can be the limiting factor in ambulation for an amputee. An individual who has a lower extremity amputation and requires a walker or crutches to ambulate uses 65% more energy than

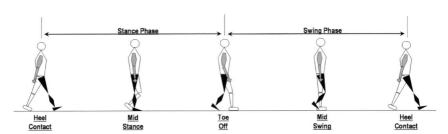

Fig. 2. Normal human locomotion. (Courtesy of Hanger Orthopedic Group, Inc., Bethesda, MD.)

an individual with two sound limbs and normal gait. Increased levels of energy consumption (percentage above normal) vary widely by amputation level, as follows [11,12]:

• Below the knee unilateral amputation—10% to 20%
• Below the knee bilateral amputation—20% to 40%
• Above the knee unilateral amputation—60% to 70%
• Above the knee bilateral amputation—greater than 200%

Energy consumption is less with a below the knee amputation than ambulating with crutches [13,14]. Ambulating with an above the knee amputation requires more energy, however, which makes the cardiopulmonary status of the patient more significant. It is essential to appreciate the specific influence of the microprocessor knee on each aspect of gait and normal activities of daily living.

Heel-strike and stance flexion

At the instance of heel contact, the momentum of the body and rotational forces acting on the knee and foot naturally forces the knee into flexion (Fig. 3). On the sound limb, the flexion moment at the knee is counteracted with a controlled quadriceps contraction to prevent the knee joint from collapsing. The knee undergoes 5° to 7° of knee flexion after heel-strike (some studies have shown that the degree of stance knee flexion can peak at 20°) [15]; this stance flexion moment serves to cushion the impact of weight bearing to the skeletal system and aids a smooth transition between swing and stance phase.

For an individual with a transfemoral amputation, there is no direct muscle connection to the knee to prevent the prosthetic knee from flexing and collapsing. With a nonmicroprocessor knee, the wearer is required to secure the knee in a safe position by actively contracting the hip extensors to "pull back" or extend the residual limb within the socket to force the prosthetic knee into extension. This motion maintains the knee in full extension and prevents it from buckling. Although this motion may prevent collapse of the knee joint, it eliminates the stance flexion motion and creates a negative

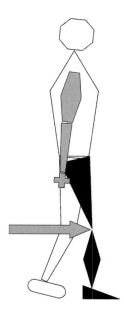

Fig. 3. Stance flexion. The moment after heel-strike, in normal gait the knee flexes 5° to 7°. This flexion serves to lessen the impact of weight bearing to reduce strain and stress to the knee, hip, and lower back. (Courtesy of Hanger Orthopedic Group, Inc., Bethesda, MD.)

influence on a normal gait pattern and can add stress to the lower back and hip joint.

The microprocessor knee monitors the rotational stress at the ankle and the flexion angle of the knee and is able to identify the moment of heel contact during the gait phase. On contact of the heel on the floor, the instant the foot starts to proceed in a plantar-flexion moment and the knee starts to flex, the continuous gait assessment function immediately (within 1/100 of a second) directs the knee electronics to adjust knee flexion resistance to provide for 5° to 7° of controlled knee stance flexion before ramping up the resistance to prevent the knee collapsing. This adjustment provides for a smooth and natural transition as the wearer bears weight onto the prosthesis when proceeding to mid-stance.

Mid-stance

At mid-stance, the prosthetic knee supports the entire weight of the wearer, and it is imperative that the knee is in the highest degree of resistance to flexion. In addition, the forces at the ankle transition from an anterior rotational moment (plantar flexion) to a posterior rotational moment (dorsiflexion). The microprocessor sensors monitor the knee flexion angle and the forces about the knee or ankle to ensure that the optimal knee flexion resistance settings are maintained to ensure the knee does not flex or collapse during this crucial phase of gait. The knee sensors also can assess a change in the weight and stress applied to the knee if the wearer picks up a heavy package. The microprocessor immediately recognizes the additional load and adjusts the knee resistance to provide greater knee flexion resistance to ensure the knee does not collapse under the combined weight of the wearer and the additional load.

Toe-off

At the instant of toe-off, the microprocessor assesses if a set of "rules" have been met and determines if the system will transition control of the knee from the microprocessor stance controller to the microprocessor swing controller. Depending on the model and style of microprocessor knee, the computer must monitor three separate criteria before the transition from stance to swing can occur: The knee must be in full extension, 20% or less of the average maximum load on the prosthesis must be applied, and the knee must have zero angular velocity. When these criteria are met, the knee recognizes that the conditions are appropriate for normal gait, and the wearer is transitioning from stance phase to swing phase.

During normal gait, the degree of heel rise and knee flexion is related directly to walking speed. For slow cadence, the knee undergoes a small degree of flexion at toe-off, and the heel lifts off the ground a small amount. At a very fast pace, the knee undergoes a much higher degree of flexion, and the heel swings up quickly and to a much greater distance. For the prosthetic wearer, when the knee transitions to the microprocessor swing control, the knee immediately reduces the resistance to knee flexion to enable a controlled and natural flexion of the knee to enable a natural and smooth heel rise from the floor. The microprocessor calculates the gait speed of the wearer based on the knee flexion speed, and it controls the degree of knee flexion to ensure the knee flexes the correct amount for the gait speed to provide an appropriate degree of heel rise.

Mid-swing

When the knee has completed the flexion motion after toe-off, it immediately transitions into an extension moment to extend the prosthetic foot forward for the next step quickly and efficiently. The microprocessor monitors and adjusts the knee's resistance to extension to ensure the knee swings forward at a speed relative to the wearer's gait speed to ensure the foot is in place for heel contact and weight bearing [16]. If the wearer is walking fast or running, the knee must swing quickly to ensure it is in the proper position for heel contact; for slower walking, the knee must swing at a lower speed.

At the end of swing phase, just before heel contact, the knee must decelerate rapidly into a fully extended position. In a sound limb, the hamstring muscles provide a controlled contraction to decelerate the extending knee, while the quadriceps maintain a contracted position to prevent rapid knee flexion at heel contact. For an above-knee amputee, these muscle groups do not have any attachment to the knee joint, and the prosthetic knee must control the knee as stance phase initiates.

The microprocessor continuous gait assessment function adjusts the knee extension damping feature, which controls the deceleration of the knee before heel-strike and establishes the criteria for the knee to convert from swing phase back to stance phase. The knee calculates the extension speed of the knee and determines the instant that it will hit 180° of full extension. Based on the knee extension angle and speed, the microprocessor ramps up the knee extension resistance to slow the knee down so that maximum resistance to extension is achieved at the moment of full extension [17]. The on-board swing phase computer ensures the knee is swinging at the appropriate speed regardless of the how often and how quickly the wearer changes walking speeds throughout the day.

When the knee is at full extension, and the force sensors identify that there is heel contact with an anterior rotational moment at the ankle, the computer recognizes that the prosthesis is entering into stance phase and transfers control of the knee over to the microprocessor stance controller.

Sitting and standing

A challenge for prosthetic wearers is that they have only one limb to lower themselves into a chair (Fig. 4). This situation adds significant stress and

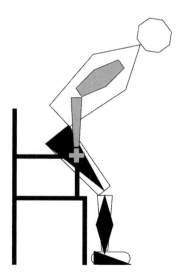

Fig. 4. Sitting and standing with a prosthetic knee. A microprocessor knee provides optimal resistance to knee flexion to reduce strain and stress to the sound side knee, enabling the amputee to lower slowly and under control into a seated position. For standing, the microprocessor knee provides no resistance to extension with maximum flexion resistance. (Courtesy of Hanger Orthopedic Group, Inc., Bethesda, MD.)

strain on the sound limb and introduces rotational forces at the hip, spine, and shoulders because the individual cannot lower himself or herself squarely into a chair using the resistance and control of two sound limbs. For a bilateral amputee wearing a nonmicroprocessor knee, sitting into and getting out of a chair are extremely difficult and precarious; in the absence of muscular control of anatomic knees and hence lacking the ability to control knee flexion actively, the individual must sit in a chair with arm rests and use upper body strength to lower into and rise from a chair. Microprocessor knees sense the motion of sitting and standing and adjust the flexion and extension resistance of the knee valves to reduce greatly strain and stress to the sound joints of the wearer and to assist in safely and securely getting in and out of a chair.

Sitting

The onboard computer senses when the wearer wants to sit down based on the posterior rotational moment at the ankle combined with the slow and deliberate knee flexion moment. The continuous gait assessment function adjusts the valves to maximum resistance of the knee to allow the wearer to "ride the knee down" to a seated position. For a unilateral transfemoral amputee, this motion greatly reduces stress and strain on the sound limb and allows the wearer to lower into the chair with even weight distribution on both feet. Bilateral amputees are able to sit into a chair without using as much of their upper body because the microprocessor sets the valves to bend with maximum knee flexion resistance, allowing the wearer to be lowered slowly and safely into a seated position. Although the microprocessor knee wearer does not require arm rests to sit into a chair, it is recommended that the wearer always choose a chair with arm rests because they are required (essential for bilateral amputees) to get up out of a chair.

Standing

While standing, the individual uses the upper body to push out of the chair, and there is a transitional moment when the individual transfers weight from the arms to a standing position, which exposes a temporary instance of instability. The microprocessor knee sensors identify the movement of standing out of a chair and set the knee so that it has little or no resistance to extension with maximum resistance to flexion. If the wearer were to lose balance while standing and put weight on the prosthesis, the knee automatically would be ready and programmed for maximum resistance and stability, preventing a fall. This is an excellent security feature for getting in and out of cars.

Stairs

An additional benefit of microprocessor stance control lies in the support it offers individuals when descending stairs step over step (Fig. 5) [18]. If an individual is to negotiate walking down stairs, the knee must provide an

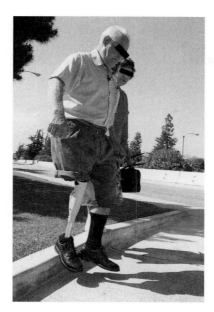

Fig. 5. Descending step with a Compact microprocessor knee. The knee sensors identify the rapid knee flexion combined with a lack of resistance at the toe and adjust the valves appropriately for maximum knee resistance to enable the wearer to descend the stair or curb safely step over step. (Courtesy of Hanger Orthopedic Group, Inc., Bethesda, MD.)

increased resistance to flexion so that the individual can descend the stairs in a controlled manner. Without muscular control of the knee joint, the wearer has limited ability to control the speed and resistance of knee flexion during weight-bearing descent of the stair. A situation is created in which the wearer must enter into a controlled fall as the prosthetic knee rapidly flexes and quickly stop the downward momentum with the sound leg. When using a mechanical prosthetic knee joint, individuals with a transfemoral amputation typically must descend stairs one at a time because it is difficult to control the flexion of the knee for safe, consistent stair descent. When descending stairs with a microprocessor-controlled knee joint, the wearer places the prosthetic foot with forefoot hanging over the step. The knee angle sensor identifies the rapid knee flexion combined with a lack of resistance at the toe and determines the need for maximum knee resistance to enable the wearer to descend the stair or curb safely step over step. The knee responds immediately to the flexion speed of the knee and external forces about the knee and foot to ensure optimal stability and function for stair descent.

Ramps and uneven terrain

Descending hills and ramps (Fig. 6) creates a significant challenge for individuals with a transfemoral amputation because of an increased knee

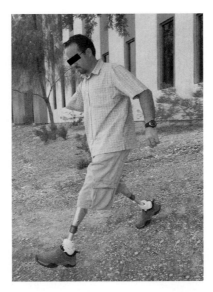

Fig. 6. Descending ramps with Otto Bock C-Leg microprocessor knee. The microprocessor quickly identifies that the prosthetic knee is descending a ramp or slope; the knee is instantaneously adjusted into ramp mode to provide optimal resistance to knee flexion and provide for a stable and secure gait for descending a ramp or slope. (Courtesy of Hanger Orthopedic Group, Inc., Bethesda, MD.)

flexion moment during stance. This increase in knee flexion is due to the increase in speed and weight transfer caused by the added momentum created by walking down a slope. When walking down a ramp, the necessary primary reaction required by the knee is to reduce the momentum and provide a controlled flexion moment at the instance of heel-strike. The microprocessor quickly identifies that the prosthetic knee is being forced into rapid flexion, and owing to the slope of the ramp, there is an absence of or delay of floor reaction to the foot. The knee is adjusted instantaneously into ramp mode to provide optimal resistance to knee flexion and provide a stable and secure gait for descending a ramp or slope. The microprocessor continuously monitors the external forces and knee position to determine if any movements are outside of normal gait patterns. If the prosthesis experiences any unexpected forces or conditions that are common while walking on uneven terrain, the computer immediately initiates the stumble recovery setting to ensure the knee is adjusted to maximum flexion resistance to ensure security and stability.

Stationary standing

When standing in a stationary position (Fig. 7) with a nonmicroprocessor knee, the wearer must maintain a focus on the position of the prosthetic

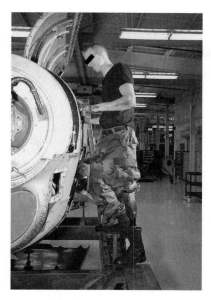

Fig. 7. Standing mode with Endolite adaptive microprocessor knee. The microprocessor recognizes that the wearer has come to standing position and adjusts itself to provide a high degree of resistance to flexion, but would allow the knee to move easily into extension. (Courtesy of Hanger Orthopedic Group, Inc., Bethesda, MD.)

knee. When standing for a long time, the body's natural response is to stand with the knee slightly flexed, but to do so with a nonmicroprocessor knee would cause the knee to go into rapid flexion and cause the individual to fall. With the microprocessor knee, the computer recognizes that the wearer has come to standing position and adjusts to provide a high degree of resistance to flexion, but allows the knee to move easily into extension. When the wearer decides to initiate gait, the knee responds within 1/50 to 1/1000 of a second and readjusts the valves for the wearer's activity and movement.

Microprocessor knee options

There are several microprocessor knee options (Table 2).

C-Leg

Although the C-Leg by Otto Bock (Otto Bock Health Care, Minneapolis, Minnesota) (Fig. 8) [6,16,18,19] is not the first microprocessor knee on the market, it arguably has set the standard with regard to the function and features for a microprocessor knee. The C-Leg uses a real-time gait analysis microprocessor to monitor the movements of the wearer 50 times/s to make instantaneous adjustments to the hydraulic valve position to ensure the knee is always in the most stable and secure settings. Although the processing

Table 2
Microprocessor knee options

	Compact	Rheo	Adaptive	C-Leg
Manufacturer	Otto Bock	Össur	Endolite	Otto Bock
Country of origin	Germany	Iceland	England	Germany
Characteristics				
Component weight	2.7 lb	3.4 lb	3.3 lb	2.6 lb
Weight limit	275 lb	200 lb	275 lb	275 lb
Stance control	Hydraulic	Magnetorheologic	Hydraulic	Hydraulic
Swing control	Hydraulic	Magnetorheologic	Pneumatic	Hydraulic
Battery	Rechargeable	Rechargeable	Rechargeable or disposable	Rechargeable
Foot options	Limited	Unlimited	Unlimited	Limited
Features				
Microprocessor stance	Yes	Yes	Yes	Yes
Microprocessor swing	No	Yes	Yes	Yes
Stance flexion	Yes	Yes	Yes	Yes
Second mode	No	No	No	Yes
Heavy duty frame	No	No	Yes	Yes
Rechargeable batteries	Yes	Yes	Yes	Yes

speed of this knee is slowest of all the microprocessor speeds, the C-Leg uses a closed hydraulic cylinder system with two valves to control the knee flexion and extension resistance. The C-Leg has the fastest reaction time to valve adjustments and always is maintained in stance control mode; it has active

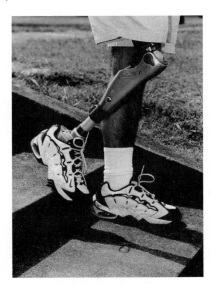

Fig. 8. Otto Bock C-Leg microprocessor knee. The Otto Bock C-Leg knee provides microprocessor swing and stance phase controls. The C-Leg is the only microprocessor knee that provides a second mode; this enables the wearer to initiate knee functions and settings for work or recreational activities in which specialized settings or movement may be required. (Courtesy of Hanger Orthopedic Group, Inc., Bethesda, MD.)

stance resistance by default. In the event the battery were to lose power, the knee automatically would position all the valves to a "safety" setting, which would enable the wearer to ambulate with the equivalent of a mechanical nonmicroprocessor knee until such time that the battery could be recharged. A 15-minute charge provides 4 hours of wearing time, and a 4-hour charge provides a full 40 hours of wearing time.

The C-Leg is the only microprocessor knee that offers the special feature of "second mode." By loading the prosthetic toe in a unique and specific pattern (it is highly unlikely that this pattern could be done accidentally), the C-Leg microprocessor changes settings from the normal first mode for everyday activities to the second mode for individuals who require unique knee settings for special activities. The microprocessor second mode can be programmed to enable the knee to perform in a specialized way (eg, as a free swinging knee for riding a bike, to lock after a few degrees of flexion for standing at a work bench for extended periods, or to stay flexed at 30° for operating heavy equipment with foot controls). Whatever the special activity required by the wearer, the certified prosthetist can program the knee to provide the optimal function in second mode.

The C-Leg uses extremely sensitive distal strain gauges that are located in the distal aspect of the attachment pylon (3–8 inches distal to the knee). Because of the sensitivity of these sensors, the C-Leg must be used in conjunction with specific feet that have been calibrated to the sensors.

Compact

The Compact knee (Fig. 9) by Otto Bock is the second generation of the C-Leg microprocessor knee. This unique knee is designed specifically for individuals who walk at slower speeds, but require the highest degree of stability and security possible for daily activities. The microprocessor monitors the movements of the wearer 50 times/s and makes instantaneous adjustments to the hydraulic cylinder valves to ensure the knee is always in the most stable and secure resistance during walking. For walking down ramps, stairs, on uneven surfaces or in the event of an unexpected stumble, the Compact knee provides the same high degree of stability as the C-Leg. During the swing phase portion of gait, the Compact knee has an internal hydraulic mechanism that enables the wearer to change speed during walking from slow to moderate speeds. The Compact knee is ideal for individuals who require the highest degree of stability but maintain a uniform walking speed and do not walk long distances on daily basis.

The Compact knee uses the same microprocessor technology and designs as the C-Leg. The Compact knee and the C-Leg are identical with regard to stability and security for stance phase. The Compact knee is a lightweight design, and the narrow body size and smooth edges provide for a well-shaped and cosmetic prosthesis. This microprocessor knee is custom designed for a specific and select prosthetic wearer. It is for the individual

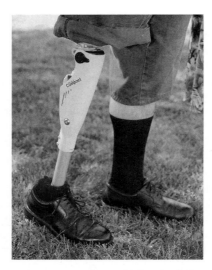

Fig. 9. Otto Bock Compact microprocessor knee. The Otto Bock Compact knee provides micro-processor stance control with manual hydraulic swing phase controls. The Compact knee is ideal for an older prosthetic wearer, who needs the highest degree of stability and security, while requiring a lower degree of variable cadence control. (Courtesy of Hanger Orthopedic Group, Inc., Bethesda, MD.)

who maintains a moderate walking speed day to day; walks on uneven ground, ramps, and stairs; and requires the highest degree of stability to prevent falls in the event of a misstep. Similar to the C-Leg, the Compact uses distally positioned strain gauges and can be used only with select feet that have been calibrated for use with this knee. In the event the battery loses power, the knee defaults to a "stability" setting, which provides for a mechanical nonmicroprocessor gait. Although the Compact uses the same battery technology as the C-Leg, it has a longer battery life because it has only a stance microprocessor controller and does not control the swing phase with a microprocessor. A 15-minute charge provides 4 hours of battery life, and a 4-hour charge provides a full 45 hours of battery life.

Adaptive

The Adaptive knee (Endolite, Centerville, Ohio) (Fig. 10) [20–22] name is appropriate because it truly describes the function of this design. The microprocessor continuously monitors each step that the wearer takes to identity changes in walking speed; ground conditions, such as uneven terrain, ramps, slopes, or stairs; and the stability of the wearer. When the microprocessor registers a change in the walking pattern, the knee automatically "adapts" to the change and adjusts the knee settings to ensure the knee is in the most stable and appropriate setting.

The Adaptive knee combines the benefits of a microprocessor-controlled knee with the stability of hydraulics and the smooth natural movements

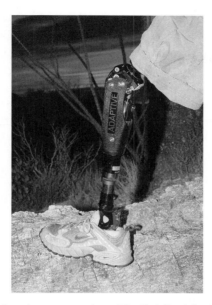

Fig. 10. Endolite Adaptive microprocessor knee. The Endolite Adaptive knee provides micro-processor-controlled hydraulic stance control with microprocessor pneumatic swing phase control. The Adaptive knee can be integrated with any style of prosthetic foot and is ideal for high-impact activities. (Courtesy of Hanger Orthopedic Group, Inc., Bethesda, MD.)

from pneumatics. For the stance phase, the knee resistance is controlled by hydraulic fluids. When the microprocessor identifies a change in the gait pattern during stance, the microprocessor adjusts internal valve settings to increase or decrease the hydraulic pressure within the knee to ensure the appropriate degree of resistance to knee flexion.

When the knee is in swing phase of walking, the microprocessor monitors and adjusts a pneumatic system to ensure the knee has a smooth and natural motion, which reduces the amount of energy used during gait. The Adaptive knee is designed and fabricated using a carbon graphite frame, and reinforced structure makes it extremely durable and able to withstand significant stress and strain. The force sensor of the Adaptive knee is located in the proximal aspect of the knee frame; although this reduces the sensitivity of the sensors, it increases the durability of the knee and eliminates the need of the prosthetic foot to be calibrated to the knee. The Adaptive knee can be used with any style or model of prosthetic foot from any manufacturer; this allows the wearer to enjoy the functions and features of prosthetic feet that may have been used on previous prosthetic devices.

For individuals who walk long distances and walk at fast speeds, the Adaptive knee provides a smooth and natural walking motion secondary to the responsive characteristics of the pneumatic swing phase control. Because the Adaptive microprocessor is continually monitoring for a *change* in the wearer's walking pattern, depending on the day-to-day activities of each individual, the battery life between charges can be 2 weeks. In addition to the rechargeable battery, there is a disposable battery option with the Adaptive knee.

Rheo Knee

The Rheo Knee (Össur, Aliso Viejo, California) (Fig. 11) [23,24] uses a unique magnetorheologic actuator and dynamic learning matrix algorithm control system. With the magnetorheologic fluid actuator, the Rheo Knee uses a magnetically influenced fluid within the knee to vary resistance (carbyl-iron spheres suspended in oil). The knee axis is a rotary design that incorporates special magnetic fluid and steel rotary blades. Resistance changes are influenced by magnetic field strength, which is controlled by a microprocessor. The knee does not use hydraulic controls for changes in resistance, but relies on changes in fluid viscosity relative to magnetic field strength and shear forces applied to the rotary blades during knee flexion and extension. Based on knee position, angular velocity, and measured loads during walking, the microprocessor determines what level of knee control is required; the microprocessor modulates the strength of the magnetic field, which changes fluid viscosity and effectively increases or decreases swing and stance resistance. The knee monitors the gait pattern at a rate of

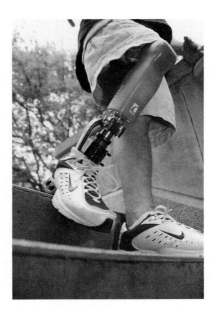

Fig. 11. Össur Rheo microprocessor knee. The Rheo Knee provides microprocessor swing and stance phase controls by using a unique magnetorheologic actuator. The knee axis is a rotary design that incorporates special magnetic fluid and steel rotary blades. Resistance changes are influenced by magnetic field strength, which is controlled by the microprocessor. (Courtesy of Hanger Orthopedic Group, Inc., Bethesda, MD.)

1000 times/s, which is necessary because the knee relies on a constant influence from the microprocessor to provide fluid viscosity changes with respect to flexion and extension resistance.

The Rheo Knee microprocessor uses the dynamic learning matrix algorithm to monitor the person's walking patterns constantly. Selected program controls rely on goals versus fixed settings. The computer targets the goal set in the computer and constantly optimizes swing phase settings to meet the goal efficiently.

The magnetorheologic actuator allows for a smooth, natural, and highly efficient gait secondary to reduced fluid drag characteristics compared with hydraulics; this allows for extremely easy initiation of knee flexion during preswing. For walking long distances or at higher walking speeds, the Rheo Knee provides effortless motion, which reduces energy consumption and provides a more natural and enjoyable walking experience.

The Rheo Knee contains strain gauge sensors in the main body of the knee and is adaptable to any style or model of prosthetic foot, allowing the wearer to enjoy the functions and features of prosthetic feet that may have been used on previous prosthetic devices. Although the Rheo Knee is the heaviest of all the microprocessor knee designs, most of the weight is from the magnetic fluid, which is distributed in the knee axis at the top of the knee. With most of the weight being located close to the knee center and close to the residual limb, combined with the smooth natural action of the Rheo Knee, there is little negative effect from functional weight of the Rheo Knee compared with other microprocessor knees.

Microprocessor knee patient selection

If an individual is unable to ambulate or lacks the ability to function with a nonmicroprocessor knee, there is little chance that he or she would be able to ambulate and benefit from the features and functions of a microprocessor knee. The microprocessor does not "create" stability, security, and function for the wearer, and it is imperative to recognize that a microprocessor knee cannot bestow ambulation and functional capabilities for the wearer. The microprocessor knee does provide, however, the wearer with the optimal degree of functional prosthetic settings and adjustments to maximize the responsiveness and reliability of the prosthesis. A detailed clinical assessment and evaluation to identify proper patient selection is essential to achieve optimal success with the microprocessor knee.

Indications for use of the microprocessor-controlled knee include the following [25,26]:

- Medicare level K3 (Box 1)—unlimited community ambulator
- Medicare level K4—active adult or athlete, who has the need to function as a K3 level in daily activities

- Select Medicare level K2—limited community ambulator. *Patient can be considered only if improved stability in stance permits increased independence, less risk of falls, and potential to advance to a less restrictive walking device, and patient has cardiovascular reserve, strength, and balance to use the prosthesis. The microprocessor enables fine-tuning and adjustment of the knee mechanism to accommodate the unique motor skills and demands of the functional level K2 ambulator.*
- Adequate cardiovascular and pulmonary reserve to ambulate at variable cadence
- Adequate strength and balance to stride to activate the knee unit
- Adequate cognitive ability to master technology and gait requirements of device
- Hemipelvectomy through knee-disarticulation level of amputation, including bilateral lower extremity amputees, who are candidates if they meet functional criteria as listed
- Patient is an active walker and requires a device that reduces energy consumption to permit longer distances with less fatigue
- Daily activities or job tasks that do not permit full focus of concentration on knee control and stability—such as uneven terrain, ramps, curbs, stairs, repetitive lifting or carrying
- Potential to lessen back pain by providing more secure stance control, using less muscle control to keep knee stable
- Potential to unload and decrease stress on remaining limb
- Potential to return to an active lifestyle

New amputees may be considered if they meet certain criteria as just outlined. Physical and functional fitting criteria for new amputees include the following:

- Premorbid and current functional assessment important
- Requires stable wound and ability to fit socket
- Immediate postoperative fit is possible
- Must have potential to return to active lifestyle

Contraindications for use of the microprocessor knee are as follows:

- Medicare level K0 (see Box 1)—no ability or potential to ambulate or transfer
- Medicare level K1—limited ability to transfer or ambulate on level ground at fixed cadence
- Medicare level K2—limited community ambulator *who does not have the cardiovascular reserve, strength, and balance to improved stability in stance to permit increased independence, less risk of falls, and potential to advance to a less restrictive walking device*
- Any condition that prevents socket fitting, such as a complicated wound or intractable pain that precludes socket wear
- Inability to tolerate the weight of the prosthesis

- Inability to use swing and stance features of the knee unit
- Poor balance or ataxia that limits ambulation
- Significant hip flexion contracture ($>20°$)
- Significant deformity of remaining limb that would impair ability to stride
- Limited cardiovascular or pulmonary reserve or profound weakness
- Limited cognitive ability to understand gait sequencing or care requirements
- Long distance or competitive running
- Patient weight or height that falls outside of recommended guidelines of manufacturer
- Specific environmental factors—such as excessive moisture or dust, or inability to charge the prosthesis

Future of microprocessor knees

The next step in integrating microprocessor technology is to provide active and functional motors to create movement, stability, and function for

---

Box 1. Medicare functional levels

K0—Lower extremity prosthesis functional level 0. Does not have the ability or potential to ambulate or transfer safely with or without assistance, and a prosthesis does not enhance the quality of life or mobility

K1—Lower extremity prosthesis functional level 1. Has the ability or potential to use prosthesis for transfers or ambulation on level surfaces at fixed cadence; typical of a limited and unlimited household ambulator

K2—Lower extremity prosthesis functional level 2. Has the ability or potential for ambulation with the ability to traverse low-level environmental barriers, such as curbs, stairs, or uneven surfaces; typical of a limited community ambulator

K3—Lower extremity prosthesis functional level 3. Has the ability or potential for ambulation with variable cadence; typical of a community ambulator who has the ability to transverse most environmental barriers and may have vocational, therapeutic, or exercise activity that demands prosthetic use beyond simple locomotion

K4—lower prosthesis functional level 4. Has the ability or potential for prosthetic ambulation that exceeds the basic ambulation skills, exhibiting high impact, stress, or energy levels, typical of the prosthetic demands of a child, active adult, or athlete

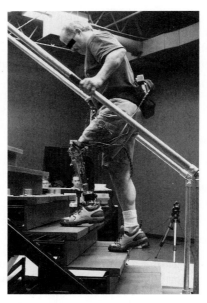

Fig. 12. Össur Experimental Microprocessor Power Knee. The microprocessor on the Össur Power Knee collects gait data from the prosthetic limb and from a stress footplate within the shoe on the sound side. The microprocessor applies advanced algorithms to assess and predict the optimal movement, position, and stability setting for the prosthetic knee and uses motors in the prosthetic knee to power the knee during gait. (Courtesy of Össur, Inc., Aliso Viejo, CA.)

transfemoral amputees. High-speed miniaturized processors are capable of collecting data from numerous sensors from the prosthetic knee and monitoring gait data from pressure-sensitive footplates inserted in the shoe of the sound side. While the prosthetic foot is in swing phase and the sound foot is in stance phase, the sensor data collected from the sound foot are transmitted to the microprocessor in the prosthetic knee. The microprocessor applies advanced algorithms to assess and predict the optimal movement, position, and stability setting for the prosthetic knee. The system applies a combination of hydraulics and miniaturized motors within the prosthetic knee to enable the wearer to walk up stairs step over step (Fig. 12). Subjects included in the early stages of development of the powered prosthesis reported reduced fatigue and performance improvement (increase in walking distance) for level ground walking. Future research will need to evaluate whether these subjective findings can be supported by objective measurement of activity and energy consumption.

References

[1] Computerized prosthesis revolutionizes treatment for amputees. Available at: www.health. uab.edu. Accessed April 1, 2004.
[2] Michael JW. Modern prosthetic knee mechanisms. Clin Orthop 1999;361:39–47.

[3] Nissen SJ, Newman WP. Factors influencing reintegration to normal living after amputation. Arch Phys Med Rehabil 1992;73:548–51.

[4] Pernot HFM, De Witte LP, Lindeman E, et al. Daily functioning of the lower extremity amputee: an overview of the literature. Clin Rehabil 1997;11:93–106.

[5] Stinus H. Biomechanics and evaluation of the microprocessor-controlled C-leg exoprosthesis knee joint. Z Orthop Ihre Grenzgeb 2000;138:278–82.

[6] Seymour R, Ordway N, Cannella P, et al. A comparison of the 3C100 C-leg prosthetic knee joint to conventional hydraulic prosthetic knees: a pilot study [abstract]. Presented at the World Confederation for Physical Therapy Fourteenth Congress. Barcelona, Spain, June 7–12, 2003.

[7] Chin T, Sawamura S, Fujita H, Nakajima S. Effect of endurance training program based on anaerobic threshold (AT) for lower limb amputees. J Rehabil Res Dev 2001;38:7–11.

[8] Flynn D. Computerized lower limb prosthesis. VA Technology Assessment Program Short Report (MDRC 152M), March 2000.

[9] Schmalz T, Blumentritt S, Jarasch R. Energy expenditure and biomechanical characteristics of lower limb amputee gait: the influence of prosthetic alignment and different prosthetic components. Gait Posture 2002;16:255–63.

[10] Traugh GH, Corcoran PJ, Reyes RL. Energy expenditure of ambulation in patients with above-knee amputation. Arch Phys Med Rehabil 1975;56:67–71.

[11] Waters RL, Perry J, Antonelli D, Hislop H. Energy cost of walking of amputees: the influence of level of amputation. J Bone Joint Surg 1976;58:42–6.

[12] Gonzalez EG, Corcoran PJ, Reyes RL. Energy expenditure in below-knee amputees: correlation with stump length. Arch Phys Med Rehabil 1974;55:111–9.

[13] Winter DA, Sienko SE. Biomechanics of below-knee amputee gait. J Biomech 1988;21:361–7.

[14] Taylor MB, Clark E, Offord EA, Baxter C. A comparison of energy expenditure by a high level trans-femoral amputee using the Intelligent Prosthesis and conventionally damped prosthetic limbs. Prosthet Orthot Int 1996;20:116–21.

[15] Fish D, Nielsen J. Clinical assessment of human gait. J Prosthet Orthot 1993;5:39–48.

[16] Kastner J, Nimmervoll R, Wagner IP. "Was kann das C-Leg?" Ganganalytischer Verleich von C-Leg, 3R45 und 3R80. Med Orthop Tech 1999;119:131–7.

[17] Datta D, Howitt J. Conventional versus microchip controlled pneumatic swing phase control for transfemoral amputees: user's verdict. Prosthet Orthot Int 1998;22:129–35.

[18] Schmalz T, Blumentritt S, Jarasch R. A comparison of different prosthetic knee joints during step over step stair decent. Orthopädie-Technik 2002;586–92.

[19] Perry J, Burnfield M, Newsam C, Conley P. Energy expenditure and gait characteristics of a bilateral amputee walking with C-Leg prostheis compared with stubby and conventional articulating prosthesis. Arch Phys Med Rehabil 2004;85:1711–7.

[20] Medical Devices Agency, Department of Health, UK. The EndoLite intelligent prosthesis. Report No. MDA/P94/03. Surbiton: Medical Devices Agency; 1994.

[21] Buckley JG, Spence WD, Solomonidis SE. Energy cost of walking: comparison of "intelligent prosthesis" with conventional mechanism. Arch Phys Med Rehabil 1997;78:330–3.

[22] Kirker S, Keymer S, Talbot J, Lachmann S. An assessment of the intelligent knee prosthesis. Clin Rehabil 1996;10:267–73.

[23] Herr H, Wilkenfeld A. User-adaptive control of a magnertorheoligical prosthetic knee. Indust Robot Int J 2003;30:42–55.

[24] Herr H, Johansson J, Sherrill D, et al. A clinical comparison of variable-damping and mechanically passive prosthetic knee devices. Am J Phys Med Rehabil 2005;84:563–75.

[25] Perlin JB. Amputee clinic teams and artificial limbs. Available at: http://www1.va.gov/vhapublications/viewPublication.asp?pub_ID = 1283. Accessed November 21, 2005.

[26] Editorial summary report: microprocessor knee patient evaluation protocol. J Prosthet Orthot 2004;16(1):31–9.

ELSEVIER
SAUNDERS

Phys Med Rehabil Clin N Am
17 (2006) 115–157

PHYSICAL MEDICINE
AND REHABILITATION
CLINICS OF
NORTH AMERICA

Orthotic Management
of the Neuropathic Limb

Nancy Williams Elftman, CO, CPed

2076 Bonita Avenue, La Verne, CA 91750, USA

Historically, the orthotist was consulted to design and fabricate devices to support or prevent deformities. As specialties arose to fulfill needs, the medical wound care community required an orthotic wound care specialty. As the wound care team and diabetes education programs develop, the outcome measures are improving, and healing times are decreasing. Multidisciplinary education programs have been instrumental in teaching all first-line caregivers to identify and monitor high-risk patients and their complications. The role of the orthotist is to redistribute weight-bearing forces by the use of custom devices for the neuropathic limb. Their role is continuous from ulcer management to accommodation and follow-up. The goal of this discipline is to prevent the first ulcer from developing when possible. The evaluation, off-loading, and prevention methods learned from orthotists have proved to be an enhancement to all wound protocols. Previously fatal outcomes have evolved into extended life spans with chronic disabilities. These complications must be monitored to avoid disability. Amputation is the complication that is most feared by diabetic patients, as many have seen loved ones lose limbs [1]. With modern wound healing techniques, risk identification, evaluation, and infection control, limb preservation is an extremely viable option [2].

Statistics

The World Health Organization estimated that the number of diabetics will increase to 366 million by 2030 [3]. Many of these individuals will not know they have diabetes until they are confronted by a life-threatening complication [4]. The prevalence of obesity and type 2 diabetes has coined the new term *diabesity*. Of all cases of type 2 diabetes, 88% to 97% are

Large portions of this article are reprinted from Elftman N. Orthotic management of the neuropathic limb. Phys Med Rehabil Clin N Am 2000;11:509–51.

E-mail address: Nancy@handsonfoot.com

1047-9651/06/$ - see front matter © 2006 Elsevier Inc. All rights reserved.
doi:10.1016/j.pmr.2005.11.002

attributed to obesity [3]. The cost of complications from diabetes is nearly $138 billion per year; amputations cost $600 million per year [5].

The estimate of adult foot problems in the United States is 50% to 80% [6]. The neuropathic (insensate) population is at a much higher risk because 40% to 50% of their foot ulcerations could have been prevented [1]. Prevention from amputation is paramount in this group. After an amputation, there is a 50% survival rate in 3 years and 40% in 5 years [1]; the contralateral limb is at risk of amputation at a rate of 50% in 4 years.

To prevent the catastrophic complications, the patient at risk must be identified. Type 1 diabetes affects siblings and children of type 1 diabetics. Type 2 diabetics generally are older than age 45 with a family history of overweight stature without exercise [4]. Both types are subject to complications after 10 to 12 years of onset. Because so many complications are seen after 12 years of diabetes, focus should include monitoring children. An increasing number of Charcot neuroarthropathy cases are reported in diabetic adolescents.

Neuropathy

Many forms of neuropathy affect the population. Neuropathy is a complication of small vessel disease. The deep tendon reflexes are affected, causing delay in motor and sensory nerve conduction [7]. These neuropathic processes cause nerve damage and the incapacity of the nerve to conduct signals of pressure and pain. Complications cause neuropathy of one or more limbs or one or more dermatome patterns [8]. Any neuropathic condition can cause paresthesia, a sensation that may range from a feeling of walking on cotton balls to pain, tingling, itching, and prickling [9].

Peripheral neuropathy

The type of neuropathy common in diabetes is peripheral neuropathy, a distal symmetric polyneuropathy. The loss of sensation commonly occurs after diabetes duration of 10 to 12 years. This complex neuropathic condition is equidistant from the spine, beginning with the feet and hands and progressing proximally to the legs and arms over time [8]. There are two major groups of peripheral neuropathy: cases that develop gradually and are usually painless or may cause numbness, burning, or "pins and needles" and cases that develop suddenly and are almost always painful, then the pain disappears.

Patients with severe pain or paresthesia may experience relief with transcutaneous electrical nerve stimulation, antidepressants, or heart medications [10]. Many medications alleviate or diminish pain, but none are known to work on large populations, and the side effects are usually undesirable. Research has been difficult to repeat in evaluating medications; one study revealed that nerve pain responded well to a placebo [8].

Trineuropathy

Peripheral neuropathy in the diabetic population involves a trineuropathy: sensory, autonomic, and motor. Sensory neuropathy is the loss of sensation, leaving the patient incapable of sensing pain and pressure. In advanced cases, the patient has no sense of identity with his or her feet and has lost the ankle jerk reflex. The level of sensation is graded by use of sensory testing protocol.

The autonomic system assists the body in maintaining a constant internal environment [11]. Autonomic neuropathy affects the sympathetic and parasympathetic nervous system. In the early stages, there may be hyperhidrosis (heavy sweating) and porokeratosis (plugged sweat glands), but late stages reveal a foot without sweat or oil production. The patient is left with dry, cracking skin that has lost elasticity and must be rehydrated constantly (Fig. 1).

Motor neuropathy is evident with the loss of intrinsic muscles. Advanced cases reveal clawing of toes and fingers (Fig. 2). The patient may experience drop foot and be prone to broken ankles and dislocated joints.

Mechanisms of ulceration

It is important to understand the cause of an ulceration to heal and prevent future breakdown. The highest incidence of ulceration is the site of a previous ulceration. A newly healed ulcer is covered with fragile skin; after

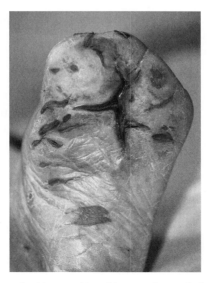

Fig. 1. Autonomic neuropathy. Dry, cracking skin secondary to lack of oil and sweat production can lead to infection.

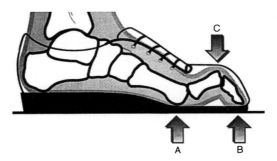

Fig. 2. Claw-toe deformity. Motor neuropathy results in loss of intrinsics and vulnerability to ulceration. (*A*) Metatarsal heads receive excess trauma because of subluxation and distal migration of fat pad. (*B*) Distal ends of toes develop callus from weight-bearing load. (*C*) Skin over dorsal interphalangeal joint receives pressure and shear forces from shoe.

complete healing, there is an area of higher density tissue (scar). The shear between different-density tissues often contributes to new ulcerations.

Mechanical stresses

Neuropathic plantar ulcers typically are roundish in shape and are caused by several different patterns of stress [12]. *Ischemic* ulcers are the result of a very low pressure (2–3 psi) over a long time. The common location of an ischemic ulcer is on the lateral fifth metatarsal head. A shoe that is too narrow for the foot produces a round ulcer as a result of depletion of blood flow at the location for a long time. *Repetitive* or *mechanical* ulcers result from normal walking pressures (40–60 psi) for thousands of repetitions per day. With normal sensation, there would be a pain signal to warn of damage to the plantar surface, but the insensate foot continues to receive the pressures as tissues weaken and become inflamed. *Traumatic* ulceration is caused by a mechanical force of very high pressure (> 600 psi) over a short period. This ulcer is the result of stepping on a piece of glass, rock, or other sharp object. Heat and chemical damage to the skin also would be categorized as a traumatic occurrence. *Infection* causes catastrophic damage with any moderate force. When an area of the foot is infected, external forces spread the infection to a greater area as pressure is applied. With any of these mechanical stresses, *shear* (pressure + friction) contributes to the breakdown process.

Chain of trauma

There is a cycle or chain of trauma with neuropathic ulcerations. The goal of the team is to break the chain before there is a permanent disability or amputation. The progression of the ulceration is as follows:

1. Trauma
2. Inflammation

3. Ulceration
4. Infection
5. Absorption
6. Deformity
7. Disability

If an ulcer is to be prevented, the foot must be protected from trauma. After an ulceration occurs, the chain must be broken as soon as possible, before infection and permanent disability.

Common complications

Constant high forces over a bony prominence can cause a *bursa* formation. A bursa often is found over the navicular (Fig. 3). Another type of bursa is a *retrocalcaneal* bursa ("pump bump") at the back of the heel caused by the use of tight shoes and high heels (Fig. 4). A neuropathic patient tends to buy shoes that are too tight to obtain sensory feedback. The bursae must be relieved of pressure before ulceration occurs.

If an ulceration is allowed to heal over at the skin level and not from deep tissues healing, there may be a pocket of bacteria trapped beneath the skin. With weight bearing, this pocket of bacteria can be spread to other tissues, causing a *sinus tract*. Another common complication for a neuropathic patient is *burns,* either by heat or chemicals, especially salicylic acid (common in corn and wart removers) (Figs. 5 and 6).

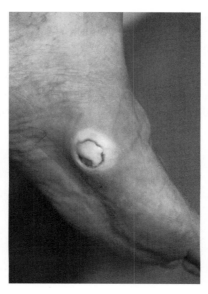

Fig. 3. Navicular bursa. Body defense owing to constant high forces over bony prominence.

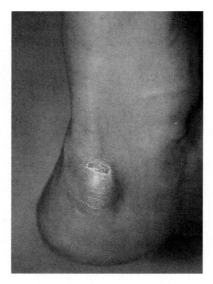

Fig. 4. Retrocalcaneal bursa (pump bump). Result of tight shoes or elevated heel.

Wound grading scales

Scales of grading ulcerations are used by orthopedic and nursing specialties; they are similar in their grading, but must be consistent within the individual clinics for consistency in charting notations. The evaluation should determine the cause of the wound and its location, its size (tracing and measurements), condition of the ulcer base (granular, fibrotic, necrotic), and the ulcer margins (undermining, adherent, macerated, nonviable) [13]. The color of the ulcer bed is noted using the Marion Laboratories wound classification (Box 1) [14].

Orthopedic specialists commonly use the Wagner Scale to classify a wound. Nurses and physical therapists use the National Pressure Ulcer Advisory Panel (NPUAP) scale [15]. These two scales are very similar (Table 1).

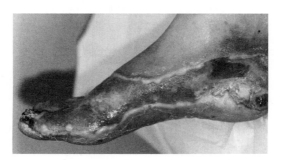

Fig. 5. Severe water burn. An insensate patient can be burned easily by hot bath water.

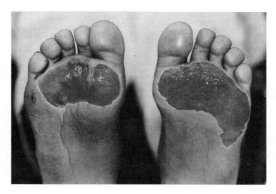

Fig. 6. Barefoot on pool deck. A neuropathic patient must wear protective shoes at all times, even around the pool.

Patient assessment

Neuropathic patients must be examined under weight-bearing and non–weight-bearing conditions. Some deformities go unnoticed until the patient walks barefoot. Because the neuropathic patient has lost sensation and motor control, the sense of proprioception also has diminished, leaving the patient to ambulate without feedback.

Leg-length discrepancy

Limb length often is overlooked during the evaluation process. The patient should be examined carefully in cases of excessive pronation or supination on one side [16]. A functional leg-length discrepancy often can be equalized with an orthosis to control the foot in a neutral position. In a structural discrepancy, an actual anatomic shortening of one or more bones, rotary changes of the spine, or the results of a surgical procedure (prosthetic hip, prosthetic knee, or fixation device) are present. Many patients have a combination of functional and structural etiology, and this combination is termed *compensation* (Fig. 7) [17].

Measurement of leg length may be obtained by the direct measurement method. The direct method requires the patient to lie supine, and a measurement is taken from the anterior superior iliac spine and distal or lateral malleolus. This method has been reported to be prone to error, however. The

---

Box 1. Marion Laboratories wound classification

Red—clean, healing granulation
Yellow—possible infection, possibly necrotic; needs cleaning
Black—necrotic, needs cleaning

Table 1
Wagner Scale and NPUAP Scale

Wagner	Description	NPUAP	Treatment goals
0	Intact skin, may be pre/post ulcer	I	Depth shoes with accommodative inserts
1	Superficial ulcer	II	Cast, splint, off-loading wound shoe*
2	Deep ulcer—full skin thickness	III	Debride, cast, splint, off-load wound shoe*
3	Extensive—muscle/ tendon/bone	IV	Remove infected tissue and improve grade*
4	Forefoot gangrene		Surgical debridement/ amputation*

* Antibiotic intervention as required.

most reliable method is the indirect technique, which requires the examiner to level the pelvic tilt with boards under the short leg to reveal the relationship between the low pelvic crest and the short leg [17].

Correcting or accommodating the leg length may be accomplished by a simple lift under the short leg. If the lift required is $\frac{1}{4}$ inch or less, the lift can be placed in the shoe. Any lift greater than $\frac{1}{4}$ inch must be placed on the sole of the shoe. The full lift should never be provided at one time, but added by $\frac{1}{8}$-inch increments. The patient's gait and pain level should improve with

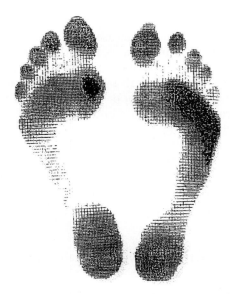

Fig. 7. Harris Mat—leg-length observance. Print is suspicious for leg-length discrepancy. Left foot has high pressures at first metatarsal head; right leg shows high pressures on lateral metatarsal head (short leg).

each added increment; if not, one should not continue to add additional height [16].

Patient evaluation should include notation of callus formation, condition of the skin, and absence of hair growth. Usually, the patient is unaware that he or she has diminished sensation, but the patient should be asked if he or she has lost feeling. If the patient has an ulceration, the patient should be asked if he or she is aware of the ulceration and what treatment has been done [18]. Many patients use home remedies for wounds, and the practitioner needs to be aware of such remedies.

Harris Mat footprints

The Harris Mat is a rubber mat developed by R. I. Harris that uses a grid pattern. The mat prints large light squares (formed by a tall grid) for light foot pressures; heavier pressures are printed in darker smaller squares (deep grid). These prints are made statically and dynamically to note the patient's compensation during ambulation (Fig. 8). The prints give a visual analysis of pressure distribution on the plantar surface of the foot and are a permanent record for the chart. The prints are used as a pattern for off-loading areas of high pressure and ulceration when a wound shoe is used during the healing process.

Semmes Wienstein monofilament (Von Frey)

The Semmes Wienstein monofilament test is a quantitative means to assess protective sensation in at-risk populations. The monofilaments are made of a brush-quality nylon monofilament. The test is performed by placing the monofilament on the skin, pressing until there is a bend or deflection, then removing the tool. This is a single-point perception test with three different diameter monofilaments to determine the patient's level of sensation (Table 2; Fig. 9).

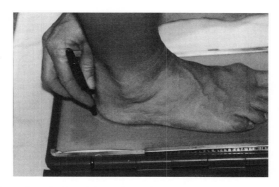

Fig. 8. Harris Mat print—heel position. The static Harris print must have posterior aspect of heel marked with a dull tool to reveal the true length for the shoe.

Table 2
Patient's level of sensation

Normal sensation	4.17 diameter	1 g force
Protective sensation	5.07 diameter	10 g force
Insensate (extreme risk)	6.10 diameter	75 g force

The monofilaments resemble needles to the patient. To calm the patient's apprehension, the clinician can show the patient the test on the hand before beginning the foot assessment. Many patients do not feel the 10 g (protective sensation) and may walk into the clinic, without a limp, on an ulcerated foot. The loss of sensation begins at the toes and progresses up the legs bilaterally (Fig. 10).

Thermometry

The use of temperature in evaluation is a quantifiable, reproducible measurement of inflammation. Inflammation is composed of redness, pain, swelling, loss of function, and heat. Although swelling and redness are difficult to grade objectively, heat is a reliable means of monitoring healing [19]. Clinicians have found the use of thermography to be simple, noninvasive, and inexpensive.

A study evaluated the effectiveness of at-home infrared temperature monitoring as a preventive tool in diabetics at high risk for lower extremity ulceration and amputation. The study group patients measured temperatures in the morning and evening and were instructed to reduce their activity and contact the study nurse when temperatures increased. This group had significantly fewer foot complications owing to their early warning of inflammation and tissue injury [20].

The temperature of the skin surface varies depending on room temperature and skin condition. On the surface of the trunk, temperatures may range from 92.3°F to 98.4°F depending on proximity to the heart. The limbs normally have equal temperatures and are symmetric. Excessive heat or coldness in one limb should signal inflammation or vascular impairment [9].

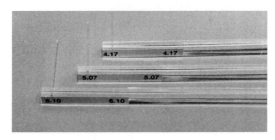

Fig. 9. Semmes Wienstein monofilament foot evaluation set. The three monofilaments for testing the foot consist of normal 4.17 (1 g), protective 5.07 (10 g), and insensate 6.10 (75 g).

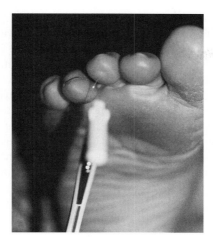

Fig. 10. Single-point perception method. Testing with monofilaments uses single-point perception. Touch the skin, deflect (bend) the monofilament, and remove. The patient should give a response when the touch is felt.

Testing begins with the patient resting with shoes and socks off for 15 minutes in a cool clinic environment. The locations for temperature measurement should be standardized for the clinic, usually six to nine plantar locations (Fig. 11). Elevated skin temperature may be predictive of future breakdown, and aggressive action should be taken to off-load the area [21]. Temperature assessment has been used to determine healing rates in surgical wounds. For the first 3 days postoperatively, the temperatures were elevated; at 4 to 8 days, the temperatures declined to show undisturbed healing of surgical site [22]. When comparing the neuropathic population,

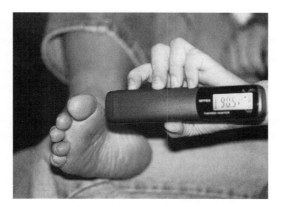

Fig. 11. Infrared thermometer. Provides thermometry method of measuring temperatures from inflammation.

neuropathy alone provided no difference in temperature of bilateral feet. Heat was a major factor in ulcerations (ulcerated area of the foot about 5.6°F higher and Charcot neuroarthropathy about 8.3°F higher) [21]. Heat defines the area of risk compared with surrounding tissue.

Diagnostic tools convert infrared radiation to a digital display to provide thermometry. The infrared thermometer not only is useful for evaluation and healing progression, but also is an excellent tool to use for follow-up. When an area of high risk has been identified, and intervention has begun, the temperatures should equalize with surrounding tissue at follow-up visits. If there is a wide discrepancy in temperatures, increased off-loading is indicated, and the patient should be examined for other complications.

Toe deformities

Although the range of motion of the ankle and hindfoot would be evaluated in standard documentation, the toes are regularly overlooked as to their importance in prevention of ulcerations. The most important toe to test is the great toe. The primary test is to dorsiflex the great toe; many neuropathic patients have a great toe that has limited or no motion at the first metatarsal head [23]. Plantar ulcerations in the neuropathic foot often are found on the first metatarsophalangeal joint (36%) as a result of atrophy of intrinsic musculature and distal migration of the fat pad [24]. The hallux rigidus deformity that limits the motion of the great toe creates high pressures as the patient walks, often resulting in an ulceration. The intervention for this patient would be a shoe with a rigid rocker bottom to enable the patient to ambulate without excessive pressures under the great toe and metatarsal head. Other deformities of the great toe include great toe pronation, which results in a plantar ulcer that extends to the outside of the great toe. This deformity can be treated with an insert that encompasses the plantar and side of the great toe. Hallux valgus (bunion) is documented as an increased angle of the great toe in relation to the first metatarsal head. Hallux extension is a hallux deformity that can be seen when the patient walks barefoot. The patient usually has callus or ulceration at the tip of the great toe at the nail because he or she thrusts the toe up into the shoe when steping. This is an uncontrolled reflex that requires a higher toe box to accommodate the excess motion.

Motor neuropathy is responsible for the loss of intrinsic control of the toes. The resultant claw toes are dorsiflexed at the metatarsophalangeal joints and plantar flexed at the interphalangeal joints. The position of the toes leaves them susceptible to trauma from shoewear by constant contact with the top of the shoe. The tips of the claw toes often show callus formation from weight bearing (Fig. 12). The distal ends of the claw toes can be relieved by assembling a custom toe crest to elevate the distal end and reduce their acquired weight-bearing function (Fig. 13). This deformity leaves the

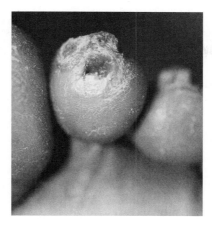

Fig. 12. Callus—distal toe weight bearing. Claw-toe deformity may result in distal tips of toes assuming weight-bearing role.

metatarsal heads with an increased load during weight bearing, causing inflammation and ulceration. When there is a prominent callus on the second metatarsal head, and the head is distal to the remaining metatarsal heads, the deformity is referred to as a Morton's toe. This condition allows the

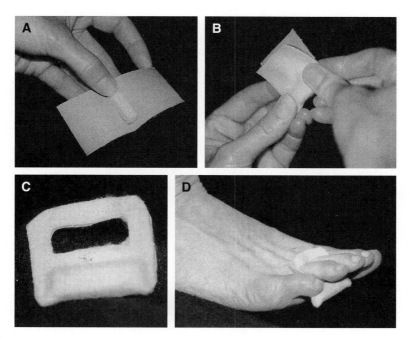

Fig. 13. Custom toe crest. Assembly is as follows: (A) Place foam on adhesive moleskin. (B) Seal foam by folding moleskin. (C) Cut opening for toes. (D) Place on toes so that foam lifts the interphalangeal joint.

second metatarsal head to receive excessive pressures from a long second or a short first metatarsal head. The area must be off-loaded and pressures spread evenly over the forefoot.

Dermatologic conditions

Some conditions of the skin require immediate attention in the clinical setting. The toes must be examined for soft corns caused by maceration. Often the maceration can be caused by not drying between the toes after bathing. To keep the area dry, the patient may use lamb's wool or tube foam between the toes. The tube foam also is used for the claw-toe deformity by reducing shear between the top of the shoe and the toes (Fig. 14). Use of the tube foam on the great or fifth toe relieves stresses with hallux deformity. Overlapping toes benefit from the tube foam application by spacing and plantar flexing the nonrigid metatarsophalangeal joint. Any corn or callus sustains increased

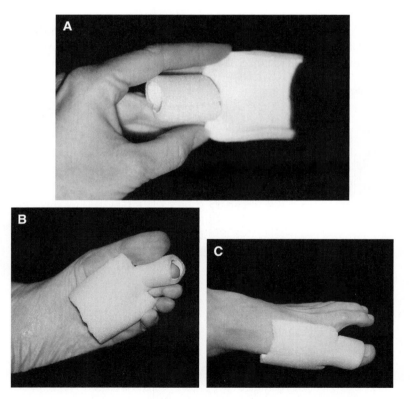

Fig. 14. Tube foam protection. The tube of foam is easily modified for use. (*A*) Make two cuts to make a "T." (*B*) Place on central toe to prevent or reduce maceration on both surrounding web spaces. (*C*) Use on great toe or fifth toe to reduce or relieve great toe bunion (hallux valgus) or tailor's bunion (fifth toe angulation).

mechanical pressure [25]. The treatment of the corns and calluses must include professional attention. Commercial corn removers are not recommended for neuropathic patients because the salicylic acid can cause chemical burns. When calluses are not reduced, they increase in thickness, become rigid, and create a shear condition with the bony prominence [20].

Skin conditions

Diabetic dermopathy (markers) are small blood vessel changes that appear in areas of light brown scaly patches on the skin. These patches do not cause pain, ulcerate, or itch [26]. Another skin change is necrobiosis lipoidica diabeticorum, which begins as a dull raised area along the tibia and evolves into a glazed scar with a violet border. Some lesions itch and are painful when they crack open [26]. Treatment is a protective dressing for the open areas of skin. Autonomic neuropathy causes the skin on the foot, especially around the heels, to become dry and crack. With the loss of sweat and oil production, the skin no longer has elasticity. This condition, keratoderma plantaris, allows keratin to build up and crack, giving small fissures that may allow an entrance for bacteria. *Pseudomonas* causes a foul-smelling localized infection with little inflammation [9]. This infection presents as a bacterial growth in a moist environment and appears green. Treatment is simply to aerate the limb and reduce the moisture.

Callus formation

Callus formation is preceded by abnormal pressure and shear. To reduce callus formation, the callus must be débrided and the abnormal forces eliminated (Fig. 15). Even when the callus has been off-loaded, it may take a considerable amount of time to break the skin's memory cycle. This concept of cellular memory in callus formation is taught in podiatry. To test this theory, a colleague studied the callus formation of patients who were comatose. To her surprise, the callus continued to form after 3 months of non–weight bearing and regular callous débridement.

Hypertrophic nails

Hypertrophic toenails must receive professional attention on a regular basis. Nails are intended to protect the ends of the toes, but are subject to trauma from shoewear and pathologic and systemic disease processes. These conditions range from ingrown nails, thick nails owing to trauma, arterial insufficiency, and fungal conditions (Fig. 16) [9].

Partial foot and toe amputations

Toe amputations may be performed surgically or by autoamputation. In many cases, the patient is not a surgical candidate, and the dry gangrene toe

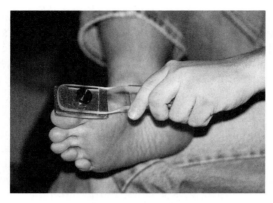

Fig. 15. Callus reduction. Callus buildup must be reduced to prevent future ulcerations second-ary to increased pressure.

eventually is autoamputated by the body. The types of toe amputations in-clude the disarticulation of the toe, toe and ray, and a full resection. When the great toe is removed, the foot must be fitted properly with a depth shoe and insole with a toe filler to prevent shear within the shoe. The second toe disarticulation allows the great toe to migrate and fill the space, creating hal-lux valgus (bunion) (Fig. 17). For this reason, it usually is recommended that second toe amputations include the ray. Amputations of central digits alone (toes 2–4) do not require a toe filler; the toe filler could cause ischemic ulcerations as the remaining toes drift to fill the resultant space, causing low continuous pressure.

The most distal amputation of the foot is the *distal metatarsal,* which leaves a long lever for ambulation. The *transmetatarsal* or *Lisfranc* amputa-tion leaves a midfoot length that usually requires a forefoot block insert and

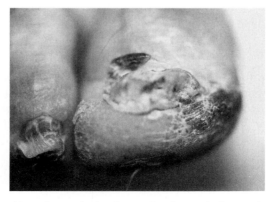

Fig. 16. Hypertrophic nails. Professional attention is required to reduce nails and treat complications.

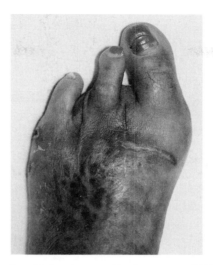

Fig. 17. Induced hallux valgus. Deformity caused by the great toe drifting to fill the space of the second toe amputation.

a high-top shoe for suspension. The *transtarsal* or *Chopart* amputation is rarely performed because it leaves a short foot that is difficult to suspend in a shoe. The *Symes* amputation results in a limb with a walking pad and can be suspended easily in a prosthesis. With all partial foot amputations, preservation of a portion of the foot retains greater ambulatory function than a transtibial amputation. The skilled surgeon balances the antagonistic muscle groups to provide a functional residual foot (Fig. 18).

Charcot neuroarthropathy

Charcot's joint is a commonly misdiagnosed and improperly treated complication in the diabetic foot. The increased skin temperature often is assumed to be an acute infection [20]. This condition involves more than one joint, so many authors refer to the complication as a Charcot's foot; incidence increases with the duration of diabetes (usually after 12 years) [2]. Although there is a higher incidence in patients older than age 40, there is no relationship between Charcot neuroarthropathy and the severity of diabetes [27]. In type 1 and type 2 diabetes, bone mass is reduced, resulting in an increased risk of fracture [28].

Dysfunction of the autonomic nervous system may be associated with Charcot's joint because the motor power to the affected joint is intact and proprioceptive impulses are diminished [29]. Autonomic neuropathy may be responsible for increased blood flow and osteoclastic activity [28]. Diabetics with neuropathy have shown significantly more radiographic abnormalities of the bone/joint structure than non-neuropathic patients. Of

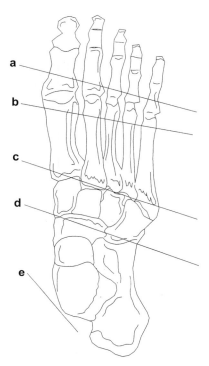

Fig. 18. Partial foot amputation levels. (*A*) Toe (distal) amputation. (*B*) Transmetatarsal amputation. (*C*) Lisfranc amputation. (*D*) Chopart amputation. (*E*) Symes amputation.

patients with previous foot ulcerations, 22% incurred traumatic fractures, and 16% revealed Charcot changes [28].

Bony fragmentation

Acute phase

The Charcot episode begins with a disassociation and destruction of joint surfaces. This is the beginning of a painless (usually) and degenerative collapse of the foot structure. The foot is swollen, red, and hot and has increased blood supply resulting in bounding pulses. Studies have shown that the blood flow is not only increased, but also grossly abnormal [3]. The presence of warmth in the early stages of Charcot neuroarthropathy may be defined easily with the use of thermography [14]. The use of infrared thermometers may be of more diagnostic use in the acute Charcot episode than standard testing methods, with local temperatures increasing by 8°F to 10°F. In the acute stage, the bones and joints begin to break down [30]. This breakdown is believed to be caused by increased activity in osteoclasts that absorb bone and decreased osteoblasts that deposit new bone. Charcot changes can occur spontaneously, but may follow a minor fracture or soft tissue injury.

Coalescence phase

In this long stage of restructure, the osteoclasts absorb the fine bony debris, and osteoblast activity increases to begin the process of bony reconstruction (Fig. 19). This stage can be monitored by the gradual decrease of temperature with the infrared thermometer. Radiographs easily define the involved area and the newly deposited bone formation with fusion of larger fragments of adjacent bone.

Reconstruction phase

The reconstruction stage is an attempt to restore the joint architecture by revascularization and remolding of bony fragments. The result of this phase is fused joint without motion, as the bony deposits mold the joint surface into a solid structure (Fig. 20). Most important to the reconstruction phase is the immobilization of the lower limb because premature return to activity can trigger another acute Charcot episode [21].

Treatment plan

The treatment plan requires immediate immobilization of the limb with the use of a total contact cast. The cast is molded to the lower limb to reduce pressures to the affected joints and spread the forces over the entire lower limb. The cast must be changed weekly until volume has stabilized, and there is no risk of movement within the cast, then cast changes may extended. This casting procedure captures the shape for the remodeling process. The Charcot limb that is not casted within the acute phase usually results in a foot with

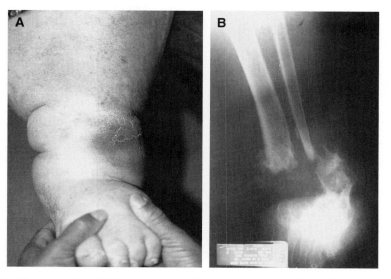

Fig. 19. Charcot ankle. (*A*) Limb is hypermobile at involved joint. (*B*) Radiograph of bony absorption.

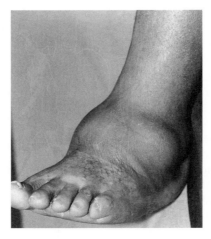

Fig. 20. Charcot hindfoot deformity. Resultant deformity requires total contact orthosis above the ankle to prevent recurrence of acute Charcot episode.

severe deformities, including a rocker-bottom foot (Fig. 21). The deformities resulting from Charcot neuroarthropathy can be difficult to accommodate in shoewear and orthoses, without recurrent breakdown.

The midfoot, especially at tarsometatarsal joints, is often involved in the destructive process and results in a rocker-bottom foot if casting is delayed

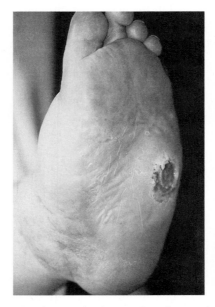

Fig. 21. Charcot midfoot. Resultant rocker-bottom foot that requires custom shoe with an accommodative off-loading orthosis or neuropathic walker.

or removed before bony reconstruction is complete. The casting can take 1 year and must be monitored carefully.

Osteomyelitis

Osteomyelitis is bone inflammation resulting from infection. Osteomyelitis and Charcot neuroarthropathy often are confused in laboratory tests and radiographs. Both conditions may have increased infrared temperatures, redness, and swelling. When there is an open access wound, and the bone can be probed, there is an 89% positive indication for osteomyelitis [18,31]. The diagnosis can be confirmed with bone biopsy when there is access to the bone. After bone destruction has been diagnosed, the bone must be surgically débrided [18,32]. Some cases of chronic osteomyelitis are not surgically débrided, but simply treated as the condition flares. The chronic condition must be followed carefully because the infection can spread. When there is no opening or wound to probe the bone, a three-phase bone scan can verify osteomyelitis by specificity, whereas MRI would measure only general sensitivity.

Vascular assessment

The patient with vascular disease must be evaluated for arterial, venous, or a combination of these conditions. The examiner begins the evaluation by a pulse examination, which includes location and grading arterial pulses on the foot at posterior tibial or dorsalis pedis arteries [15]. The grading system for pulses is shown in Table 3. The standard grading for pitting edema of the lower leg is shown in Table 4.

Ankle/brachial index

The ankle/brachial index (ABI) supplies objective information as to the presence of arterial occlusive disease. The values are obtained by the use of a Doppler probe (ultrasound stethoscope, blood pressure cuff, and ultrasound gel). The highest ankle Doppler pressure is divided by the highest brachial Doppler pressure to determine the ABI. The values obtained assist the practitioner in assessing the patient (Table 5). Ischemia determines the ability of the diabetic foot to heal. With advances in vascular surgery, many

Table 3
Pulse grading system

0	No pulse
1 +	Barely felt
2 +	Diminished
3 +	Normal pulse (easily felt)
4 +	Bounding pulse

Table 4
Grading for pitting edema of the lower leg

0–$\frac{1}{4}$ inch pitting	1 + (mild)
$\frac{1}{4}$–$\frac{1}{2}$ inch pitting	2 + (moderate)
$\frac{1}{2}$–1 inch pitting	3 + (severe)
>1 inch pitting	4 + (very severe)

Data from Sandrow RE, Toro JS, et al. The use of thermography in the early diagnosis of neuropathic arthropathy in the feet of diabetics. Clin Orthop 1972;88:31–3.

patients may have improved ABI status after vascular reconstruction, which improves the outcome and decreases the incidence of amputation [33].

Arterial disease

Atherosclerosis is the hardening of the arteries. The smooth interior walls of the arteries become layered with platelets, calcium, and connective tissue deposits; severe obstruction depletes flow to distal extremities (Fig. 22). With advanced disease, the arteries are visible on radiographs. Arterial disease is painful and aggravated by elevation [34]. An important test is for dependent rubor, which occurs when the leg is elevated causing blanching of the limb [35]. Other arterial characteristics include the following:

Foot cool/cold
Weak or absent pulses
Absence of leg hair
Skin shiny, dry, pale
Ulcer below ankle/necrotic with minimal drainage
Ulcer appears "punched out" without bleeding

Venous insufficiency disease

Venous insufficiency is caused by calf and muscle pump failure [34]. An obvious venous complication is varicose veins, which are dilations of peripheral veins with discoloration [9]. Failure of the venous pumping system causes edema, which represents water and sodium buildup. Venous stasis ulcers are caused by venous hypertension and an increase in capillary

Table 5
Ankle/brachial index values

ABI value	Significance
>1	Referral to vascular specialist. Indicates calcified vessels if diabetic
0.8–1	Venous insufficiency. Mild arterial disease (compression therapy)
0.5–0.8	Referral to vascular specialist. Intermittent claudication indicates peripheral arterial occlusive disease (compression contraindicated)
<0.5	Referral to vascular specialist (compression contraindicated)

Data from Sussman C, Bates-Jensen BM. Wound care: a collaborative practice manual for physical therapists and nurses. Gaithersburg (MD): Aspen Publishers; 1998.

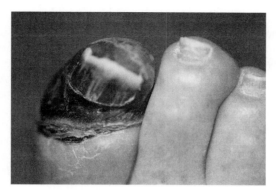

Fig. 22. Arterial insufficiency. In severe arterial disease, dry gangrene may result from insufficient blood supply.

pressures (Fig. 23) [36]. Characteristics of venous disease include the following [14]:

Warm foot
Edema
Skin pigment changes
Varicose veins
Ulcer not usually painful, has granulation and drainage
Ulcer location above ankle (anteromedial malleolus)

Compression therapy

The pooling of fluids in the lower leg does not allow delivery of new oxygenated blood. The treatment for edema is graduated compression when the ABI indicates a venous disorder. Before compression therapy can be considered, the ABI must be obtained to ensure that there is no compression applied to a lower extremity with arterial disease. With an ABI greater than

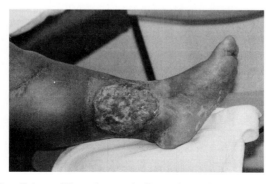

Fig. 23. Venous insufficiency. Ulcerations typically are located anteromedial malleolus owing to thin skin and proximity of veins to the skin surface.

0.8, the treatment would be compression of 35 to 40 mm Hg with graduated compression because this would be a limb with venous insufficiency. An ABI of 0.6 to 0.8 can be compressed only with 20 to 25 mm Hg owing to arterial and venous insufficiency. Any ABI less than 0.6 mm Hg is compromised by arterial disease and is compromised further by compression. A limb with an ABI less than 0.45 is not likely to heal from an ulceration or amputation and is at extreme risk.

The leg with a venous stasis ulceration must be elevated above the heart level, especially in the afternoon, to counter the effect of gravity on pooling fluids. The periodic elevation decreases pressure against the expanded vein wall [9]. The leg must be dressed with appropriate wound care protocol and wrapped with one of the many compression therapy applications on the market. Unna's boot also may be used over the dressing. Unna's boot is a zinc oxide compression wrap that protects vulnerable skin from weeping exudate distal to ulcerated tissue (Fig. 24). This semirigid dressing is a combination of gelatin and zinc oxide that is applied wet. As the wrap dries, it becomes a nonexpandable, nonshrinkable porous mold. The edema is controlled by crossing the ankle joint and allowing motion of the joint and musculature to generate a pumping motion for the lower extremity.

Pressure gradient stockings

The lower limb with chronic venous insufficiency can be controlled with pressure gradient stockings that assist in the function of distended veins. The compression begins distally and is reduced proximally to resist backflow caused by defective venous valves (Fig. 25). The stocking is most effective below the knee to facilitate the pumping action. For all stockings, the practitioner must measure the patient in the morning when the limb is at its lowest volume. Each stocking manufacturer requires specific measurements and offers different options for their product. In severe cases, the limb should be

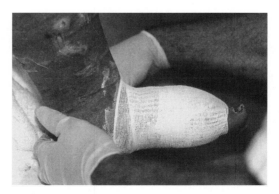

Fig. 24. Unna's boot. Application of this zinc oxide compression wrap begins at metatarsal heads and continues past the calf.

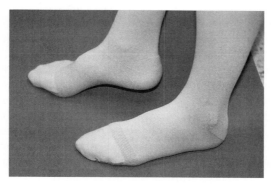

Fig. 25. Pressure gradient stocking Compression begins at the foot and decreases proximally to assist in pumping function of musculature.

pumped or wrapped before measurements are taken. A neuropathic patient should never have seams in the area of a bony prominence (metatarsal heads, malleoli, heel). If the edema includes the foot, the patient requires full foot compression to begin the pumping action at the metatarsal heads, the most distal level. The compression stockings also are used to modify and reduce scarring and shape a residual limb after amputation [17]. The antiembolism stocking is designed to be worn by patients confined to a hospital bed to help prevent blood coagulation. These stockings are not designed to counter the gravitational pooling when ambulating. The antiembolism compression is approximately 18 mm Hg and stimulates blood flow only. Compression stockings range from 20 to 30 mm Hg to greater than 60 mm Hg. The compression classes of stockings are shown in Table 6.

In all cases of venous insufficiency, both legs should be monitored. If one leg has had a venous ulceration, the other leg may begin to show signs of "weeping" fluids. Control of both extremities is important in the use of compression stockings. No pressure should be used in cases of infection or woody (fibrous) edema because the limb cannot be compressed.

Table 6
Compression classes of stockings

Class I	20–30 mm Hg
	Light venous insufficiency, mild edema, mild varicose veins
Class II	30–40 mm Hg
	Moderate venous insufficiency, post-thrombosis, severe variscosities, healed venous ulcer
Class III	40–50 mm Hg
	After treatment of severe ulcerations, severe chronic venous insufficiency, lymphedema
Class IV	>60 mm Hg
	Severe edema, open ulcer, lymphedema, elephantiasis

Compartment syndrome

A compartment syndrome can occur as a result of the accumulation of fluid at high pressure within a closed muscle compartment [37]. This condition can be caused by circular plaster casts and after any fracture that has bleeding and swelling. The compartment space is determined anatomically by an unyielding fascial and bony enclosure [9]. The patient experiences diffuse tightness and tenderness owing to the pressure that obstructs venous outflow causing further swelling. The symptoms of compression on a peripheral nerve affect the motor, sensory, and autonomic functions of the nerve [9]. By reducing swelling in the limb with induced compartment syndrome, many patients experience return of sensation.

Shoes

The importance of proper shoewear and design is the basis of long-term neuropathic foot treatment and prevention of ulcerations. The shape of the shoe (last) must match the foot to reduce the possibility of high pressure points (Fig. 26). The purpose of therapeutic footwear is for long-term redistribution of weight-bearing forces for a neuropathic foot; therapeutic footwear should not be used for wound healing [38]. The shoe should be constructed of soft leather without seams over bony prominences. The leather conforms to the shape of the foot or can be stretched easily for extreme prominences (Fig. 27). Improperly tanned leathers may produce burning for the patient [9]. Neuropathic patients should be monitored for dermatologic complications because they do not have the feedback information required.

The sole of the shoe should be shock absorbing and easily modifiable for accommodating deformities. The most common sole modification is the rigid rocker sole, which allows ambulation with reduced pressures on the forefoot. This modification requires an addition to the sole thickness with an apex at 1 cm proximal to the metatarsal heads for the foot to roll over the forefoot.

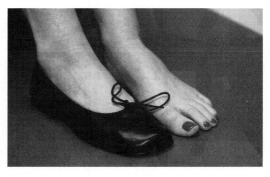

Fig. 26. Matching the shape of the shoe to the foot. The shape (last) of the shoe must be chosen to match the foot shape and characteristics.

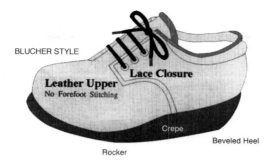

Fig. 27. Therapeutic shoe. The therapeutic shoe for neuropathic and high-risk patients provides an upper construction that conforms to the patient's foot and sole construction to reduce trauma to joint structures.

The purpose of any modification for the neuropathic foot is to allow the ground to match the weight-bearing surface of the foot, rather than to add corrections. Correction methods apply forces that cause ulcerations because the neuropathic foot cannot respond to the pressure feedback they are supplying.

The sizing of shoes is paramount, regardless of the measuring device used. The length of the shoe must be ½ to ¾ inch beyond the longest toe to accommodate the natural elongation of the foot during ambulation. The length of the shoe and the "arch length" are important (Fig. 28). The arch length is measured at the metatarsal heads and ensures that the shoe bends at the same area as the foot's bending motion. It is wise to use a shoe with the correct arch length, even if the shoe is too long. For a foot that does not match the arch and foot length requirements, a shank and rocker bottom can be used to fulfill the patient's requirements. The width of the shoe must accommodate the foot at the metatarsal heads. For a patient with proprioception or slight drop foot, addition of nonshear material to crepe soles reduces the incidence of the toe "catching" on carpet (Fig. 29). Neuropathic patients always request small shoes because they require high pressures to "feel" the shoes. These patients must be fitted by a professional; patients must break the shoes in by wearing them 2 hours per day with increased time each day. Sandals are not recommended as shoewear because of the strap shear and incidence of damage to toes from the external environment. Shoes with laces provide the most control over the forefoot, but many patients have neuropathy in the upper extremities or visual impairment, which requires the conversion of the shoe to Velcro or other methods of closure.

Accommodative insoles

Patients without protective sensation must be accommodated with insoles in their shoes. Depending on the amount of off-loading of bony prominences, the shoe must have enough depth to contain the insole and the foot deformity. For a neuropathic foot, the multidensity insole materials should be

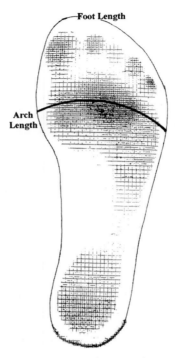

Fig. 28. Shoe sizing. The shoe length should be ½ inch to ¾ inch beyond the longest toe. The arch length determines the "bend" of the shoe, which must match that function on the foot.

compressible by half of the full thickness to allow for deformation through the gait cycle. The upper layer that contacts the foot should be a material that is closed cell and self-molding to allow the foot to mold the material further. The middle layer should contain any padding (metatarsal pads, scaphoid pads) and be shock absorbing (poron, microurethanes), and the base should support the foot structure securely (Fig. 30). The insole and shoe must be replaced when wear prevents the optimal function of either. The shoe and insole must be inspected daily for wear and foreign objects. Wear patterns should reveal possible modifications necessary for the current shoe/insole combination and future design requirements. Follow-up of the patient should include temperature testing to determine if the off-loading has been effective. Increased temperatures after 2 weeks indicate a need for additional off-loading.

Toe fillers and toe and forefoot blocks

Ideally, a patient with a partial foot should wear a short custom shoe, but noncompliancy and cosmesis usually dominate, and the patient selects a full-size shoe with a block to replace the missing foot section. The toe or forefoot blocks reduce migration of the foot within the shoe and support

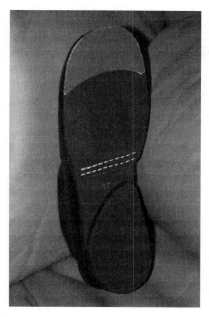

Fig. 29. NonShear toe. Reduces "catching" toe on carpet with crepe soles.

the dorsal shoe structure. Central digit amputations should not be spaced with toe fillers because there is a probability of ischemic ulcerations owing to the drifting of remaining toes. Forefoot blocks impinge on the distal end of partial foot amputations without a rocker bottom of the shoe or a "toe break" in the insert where the shoe normally would bend dorsally.

Socks

Socks for neuropathic limbs should have no seams over bony prominences and no mended areas. A blend of materials helps wick away perspiration

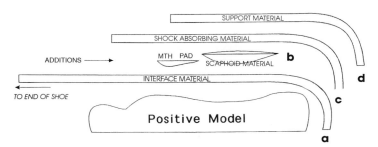

Fig. 30. Accommodative insert fabrication. The accommodative insole is fabricated over a positive cast model of the foot by layers: (A) Interface material. (B) Necessary pads: metatarsal or scaphoid. (C) Shock absorption material. (D) Semifirm support material.

to maintain a dry environment. Socks should have nonrestrictive calf open-ings and be used to try on shoes for optimal fitting (Fig. 31). Technology today has offered many options in sock construction and function. The par-tial foot now can be accommodated with a sock that does not have seams over the distal end; the toe sock allows air between toes to eliminate macer-ation and reduce toes overlapping. There are many diabetic/neuropathic socks available with nonrestrictive tops and minimal or no seams over bony prominences. The patient is instructed to use white or a light color next to the foot to allow immediate recognition of drainage. The sock plays an important roll in breaking in the new shoe and orthosis. The use of two thin socks instead of one thick sock assists in reducing blisters caused by shear as the shoe is slowly molding to the foot.

Custom ankle-foot orthoses

Many neuropathic deformities can be controlled only by crossing the an-kle joint to reduce plantar pressures. These chronic deformities include chronic ulceration, Charcot deformity, and hindfoot/ankle deformities. The ankle-foot orthosis is required when shoes, modifications, and insoles cannot reduce the occurrence of breakdown. All neuropathic custom devices are casted semi–weight bearing on a foam pad to capture the exact structure of the foot's plantar surface. If the patient is not semi–weight bearing, the forces that are normally applied are not reflected in the positive model.

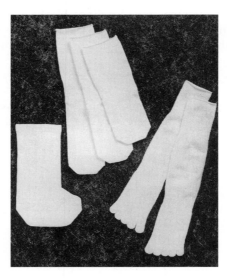

Fig. 31. Specialty socks for the neuropathic foot. The neuropathic foot requires wrinkle-free, seamless socks that wick away perspiration and reduce maceration. Socks are designed to meet the needs of the partial foot, full neuropathic foot, and foot with toe complications, especially maceration between toes.

Total contact ankle-foot orthosis

The total contact ankle-foot orthosis is a custom orthosis that distributes weight-bearing forces over the entire lower leg to minimize peak pressures on the plantar surface. This orthosis is formed over the custom lower leg cast and contains a full lining and a total contact insole. The orthosis must be fitted into a shoe, which makes the donning complicated.

Neuropathic walker

The neuropathic walker (also referred to as charcot restraint orthotic walker [CROW]) is casted and prepared in the same manner as the total contact ankle-foot orthosis, but it totally encloses the limb with plastic, lining, and removable insole (Fig. 32). The design of this walker locks the ankle to reduce force through the Lisfranc joint or ankle. The removable insert can be formed over any chronic breakdown area, including medial or lateral malleoli (Fig. 33). The advantage of the walker is that the sole does not require a shoe. The sole of the neuropathic walker is a rocker bottom and designed to replace the additional shoe.

Axial resist or patella tendon bearing orthosis

The patella tendon bearing orthosis is intended to decrease forces on the plantar weight-bearing surface of the foot. This design has been used successfully for partial calcanectomy, plantar skin graft, and heel ulceration patients. This orthosis decreases, but does not eliminate, weight-bearing forces

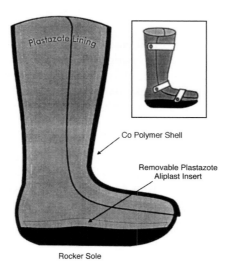

Fig. 32. Neuropathic walker (also known as "CROW"). The custom total contact walker provides ambulatory security for severe deformities that cannot be accommodated in therapeutic footwear.

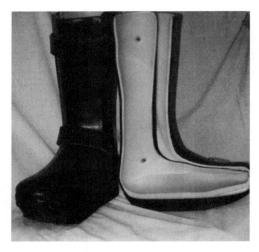

Fig. 33. Total contact interface. Interface reduces shear to high-risk skin. Insole is removable to accommodate changes in pressure areas.

by circumferential forces below the knee. The orthosis is contraindicated for patients with compromised vascular status because of the pressures on the popliteal artery that could impinge on arterial flow.

Off-loading ulcerations with ankle-foot containment

In the treatment of any ulceration, there must be wound care protocol with cleansing, dressing, and off-loading of the affected area. This combination has shown optimal results in the healing of wounds and requires a team to be involved. Prefabricated and custom applications are available for the clinical team to consider for each patient. Many patients are given crutches, walker, or wheelchair, but may not have the upper body strength, cardiovascular reserves, or motivation to use assistive devices [38]. Bed rest eliminates the pressures on the foot, but promotes deconditioning of the patient [39].

Prefabricated ankle-foot orthoses

The simple reinforced foam ankle-foot orthosis is employed most often for night use. There are several types on the market that reduce contractures by retaining the ankle position in neutral. These devices also are used for heel ulcerations that break down secondary to low ischemic pressures over long periods.

Prefabricated walkers

Prefabricated walkers are commonly used for severe ankle sprains and foot/ankle fractures. They are convenient, lightweight, and removable with fixed ankle joints and a rocker sole [40]. With the semirigid shell, they may be reused for future breakdown, which makes them cost-effective [38]. The purpose of the walker is to reduce the amount of time spent on a bony prominence by limiting movement of the tibia on the talus to reduce plantar flexion and dorsiflexion [24]. Many walkers provide methods of filling the space around the limb, but they are not total contact devices. Low-risk patients are usually candidates for this method of off-loading.

Posterior splint

The posterior splint is not an off-loading device, but an excellent transition from a total contact cast method of off-loading to use of shoes. The posterior support is not circumferential to off-load the plantar surface, but can reduce pressure to an ulcerated area with inclusion of an off-loading plantar insole.

Total contact cast

The total contact cast has been the "gold standard" for healing ulcerations and decreasing deformity from Charcot neuroarthropathy. The cast is the most frequently cited method of reducing vertical forces per unit area. The application of the total contact cast requires training and experience in the method to prevent further injury to the compromised limb [38]. When properly applied, the cast moves plantar forces to leg shearing forces to protect pressure areas [41]. The cast controls edema, protects the limb from further trauma, and keeps the wound dry and clean. The pressures at a plantar ulceration site can be reduced by 76% by total contact casting [39]. Contraindications for use of a healing cast are shown in Box 2 [41]. The cast must be changed after 1 week because of volume reduction and subsequently changed weekly until volume has stabilized and there is no movement within the cast.

Orthotic Dynamic System splint

The Orthotic Dynamic System (ODS) splint was designed to be used in a large variety of lower extremity ulcerations. This custom orthosis accommodates edema; high-risk limbs; and wounds requiring daily monitoring, cleaning, or dressing changes [42]. The casting method is similar to the total

---

Box 2. Contraindications for use of a healing cast

Infection: redness, swelling, warmth, fever
Hypertrophic skin: thin, shiny appearance, dermatitis
Marked dependent edema
Wound size greater in depth than width (healing may seal at skin
    margins, creating a sinus tract

contact cast except there is more padding, and it includes an integral accommodative insole (Fig. 34). The ODS splint is made of fiberglass and is bivalved for daily inspection and wound care. The fiberglass construction allows the patient to ambulate within 30 minutes of application (Fig. 35). The locations that can be treated with the splint include plantar surface, heel, medial or lateral malleoli, and Symes (weight-bearing surface). When the insole is made, the material is formed over the ulcerated area with minimal dressing thickness. The insert remains full thickness and is placed on the limb to be included in the casting. After the splint is bivalved, the insert is modified to reduce pressures at the ulcer site. The insert may be removed and modified as necessary to accommodate off-loading of the ulceration. The volume changes in the limb usually can be accommodated by the addition of socks to retain total contact [42].

Off-loading plantar surfaces—specialized shoes

There are inexpensive alternatives for off-loading ulcerations with wound care protocol. In a wound care market that was expected to grow to $2.57 billion by 2002, the protocol for wounds must include methods that decrease healing times and provide an optimal healing environment [43]. For a neuropathic ulcer to heal, repetitive pressure must be reduced or eliminated by external devices. Treatment of ulcerations should focus on keeping the patient

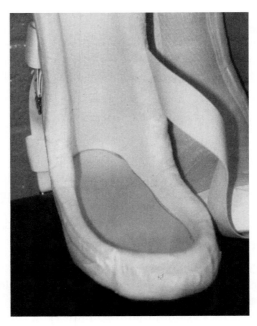

Fig. 34. ODS splint. The ODS splint has an integrated off-loading insert that is fully adjustable for areas of ulceration and high risk.

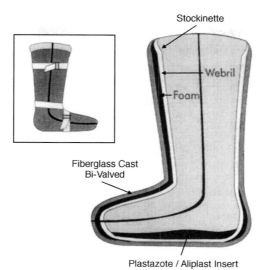

Fig. 35. ODS fabrication. The splint is fiberglass with a well-padded lining. Volume of the limb is accommodated with sock management.

ambulatory as a productive member of society [38]. More than one third of patients seen by home care practitioners have wounds. There is a low use of specialty dressings and off-loading devices in home care, and the methods are usually "clean" instead of "sterile" [44]. Introduction of off-loading devices would enhance the home care protocol. All of the following off-loading shoe devices would be improved in function by the addition of a custom accommodative insert. The area of off-loading can be designed using the patient's Harris Mat footprint as a pattern. Follow-up appointments should include temperature measurements to ensure proper off-loading. If the temperatures have increased, the off-loading area must be increased; if the temperature differential is lower, the wound is healing [21].

Plastazote healing sandle

The healing sandle contains a molded foot bed and has a rigid rocker sole. The device is lightweight, but requires considerable time and experience to fabricate [38]. This is an excellent off-loading device, but does not control movement of the foot. The sandle has been used as an interim device before definitive footwear [6].

Half shoes

Many clinics use the "half shoe," which suspends the ulcerated area, providing complete off-loading of the ulceration area. The forefoot half shoe provides a pressure-free area for the forefoot and especially the common hallux ulcerations. The heel relief shoe suspends the heel for noncontact healing. These devices may be contraindicated for a patient with limited ankle motion or balance problems associated with proprioception. Assistive devices may be required to reduce the incidence of falls [38,39].

Wedged shoes

The wedged shoe has full contact with the foot, but reduces load by reducing the amount of sole in contact with the ground. The sole angle is designed to shift weight bearing away from the ulcerated area. Patients with limited range of motion and poor proprioception may not be able to ambulate without assistive devices.

Postoperative and cast shoes

Many facilities use inexpensive postoperative shoes (rigid soles) and cast shoes (roller soles) to contain the ulcerated foot. These shoes keep the foot off the ground and allow for the bandage volume, but do not offer an intimate fit to control foot motion [25]. Most foot accommodation requires modification of Velcro straps. Without other devices available, the postoperative or cast shoe may be modified to reduce ulceration pressures, but must be monitored carefully.

Wound shoe

The wound clinic requires an immediate off-loading device to accommodate the wound care protocol. With minimal experience, the wound care practitioner can provide a dressing and an off-loading device at the time of wound dressing. The shoe has a well-padded accommodative upper with state-of-the-art closure to control foot motion. The off-loading technique reduces pressure and shear at the ulcer site through the healing process and can be modified or enhanced at any time. The rocker sole and beveled heel provide immediate ambulation (Fig. 36). The shoe was developed to contain the complete materials required for off-loading ulcerations on the plantar or heel surface (Fig. 37).

Preparation of the off-loading insole

The most important addition to the dressing and wound healing shoe is the off-loading insole that is intimately fitted to the foot. The pattern for the insole is fashioned from the static Harris Mat print that shows the area of ulceration. The heel mark should correspond to the most posterior prominence of the heel, not the Harris print (Fig. 38). The relief for an ulcerated area should be an elongated oval to allow for the normal ½ to ¾ inch excursion pattern of the foot; a circle relief would cause irritation to the healing area by constant irritation of the wound. Using the Harris pattern, the top layer remains solid, and the underlying layer contains the relief (Figs. 39 and 40). The material that interfaces with the foot should be solid without

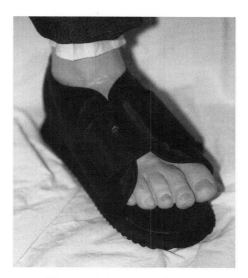

Fig. 36. Clinical wound shoe. The wound shoe is made for the left or right foot and has a new state-of-the-art closure design to control foot motion while off-loading the area of ulceration.

cutouts and heated to provide a custom contact surface. All relief areas must be on the underlying material to reduce pressures indirectly. The off-loading insole is adhered to a cast or postoperative shoe (Fig. 41). The wound shoe accommodates the insole without adhesives.

Documentation

Documentation of subjective and objective information is invaluable for historical and follow-up procedures. An excellent method of ulceration recording is with transparent film (radiographic). The tracing documents ulcer margins and callus area around the perimeter. Each follow-up visit is recorded on the same film to show healing progression. The patient is given a tracing to

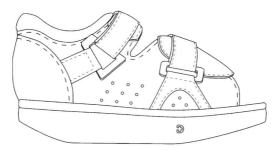

Fig. 37. Wound shoe. Well-padded shoe to allow immediate off-loading of ulcerations in the clinical setting.

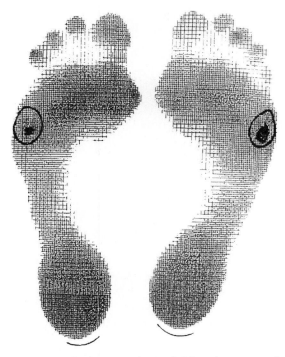

Fig. 38. Harris print as off-loading pattern. The Harris Mat print serves as the off-loading pattern in conjunction with wound care protocol. The mark at the posterior heel designated the most posterior margin to judge exact relief area. Reliefs to off-load ulcerations are elongated ovals to reduce leading edge shear.

allow him or her to see progression at home. This method of patient involvement has increased compliancy with wound care. Other objective information to be recorded is the temperature assessment and monofilament sensory test. The most useful documentation is with photographs to show the depth and granulation of the wound. The documentation protocol of the practitioner must remain consistent and contain all follow-up information (Fig. 42).

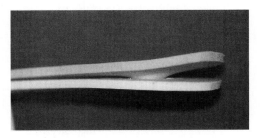

Fig. 39. Off-loading insole assembly. The material that interfaces with the foot is always solid. The underlying material is skived to off-load the ulceration.

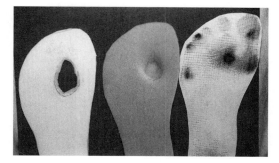

Fig. 40. Off-load molding. Heating the insole materials begins the molding process; weight and body heat continue the total contact mold.

Patient education

The education of patients and family members promotes healing and prevention of future breakdown complications. The patient must be instructed to inspect the foot daily with mirrors, magnifying glass, and family members. Footwear and orthoses should be inspected for foreign objects and areas of wear. Burns are a common complication that can be prevented by testing water before bathing, wearing water shoes on pool decking, and avoiding use of heating pads and hot water bottles. The patient should

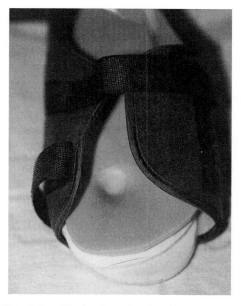

Fig. 41. Temporary off-load shoe. The insole can be placed in a cast or postoperative shoe with adhesive. The wound shoe requires no adhesive for placement.

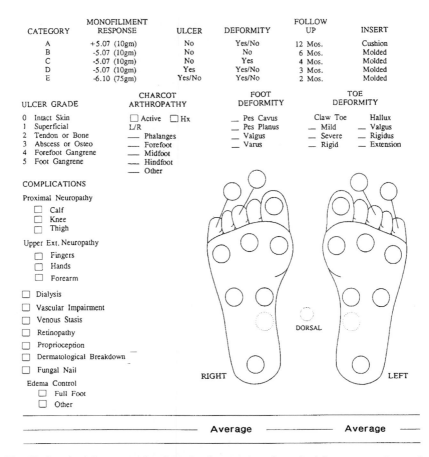

CATEGORY	MONOFILIMENT RESPONSE	ULCER	DEFORMITY	FOLLOW UP	INSERT
A	+5.07 (10gm)	No	Yes/No	12 Mos.	Cushion
B	-5.07 (10gm)	No	No	6 Mos.	Molded
C	-5.07 (10gm)	No	Yes	4 Mos.	Molded
D	-5.07 (10gm)	Yes	Yes/No	3 Mos.	Molded
E	-6.10 (75gm)	Yes/No	Yes/No	2 Mos.	Molded

ULCER GRADE

0 Intact Skin
1 Superficial
2 Tendon or Bone
3 Abscess or Osteo
4 Forefoot Gangrene
5 Foot Gangrene

CHARCOT ARTHROPATHY

☐ Active ☐ Hx
L/R
___ Phalanges
___ Forefoot
___ Midfoot
___ Hindfoot
___ Other

FOOT DEFORMITY

___ Pes Cavus
___ Pes Planus
___ Valgus
___ Varus

TOE DEFORMITY

Claw Toe   Hallux
___ Mild   ___ Valgus
___ Severe   ___ Rigidus
___ Rigid   ___ Extension

COMPLICATIONS

Proximal Neuropathy

☐ Calf
☐ Knee
☐ Thigh

Upper Ext. Neuropathy

☐ Fingers
☐ Hands
☐ Forearm

☐ Dialysis
☐ Vascular Impairment
☐ Venous Stasis
☐ Retinopathy
☐ Proprioception
☐ Dermatological Breakdown
☐ Fungal Nail

Edema Control

☐ Full Foot
☐ Other

Average ———————   Average ———

Fig. 42. Standard documentation form. Implementation of standard form to record sensation, temperatures, ulcerations, deformities, and follow-up.

never use medicated corn pads, which can lead to chemical burns. Autonomic neuropathy prevents the elasticity and leaves the skin dry. Any adhesive product (eg, Band-Aids, tape, pads) removes a layer of skin when it is removed (Fig. 43). Dehydrated skin is especially susceptible to trauma. The foot should be washed with nondrying soap and towel dried, especially between the toes. Petroleum jelly or lanolin should be applied to retain the natural moisture and covered with a sock before bed [45].

Teaching patients to remove their shoes when they eat ensures that the foot is not subjected to low pressures over a long time and reduces incidence of ischemic ulcerations, especially over the lateral fifth metatarsal head. Patients have many questions when dealing with complications. Attendance and education of other disciplines prepare the practitioner to guide the patient to the proper authority or specialty.

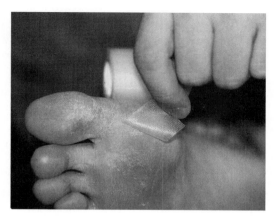

Fig. 43. Patient education. Patients and clinical personnel must be instructed in the use of adhesives. In the presence of autonomic neuropathy, any adhesive (eg, Band-Aid, tape, pads) is contraindicated. The dehydrated skin would be damaged when adhesives are removed.

Summary

The most common complaint of neuropathic patients is that they were unaware of the neuropathic pathway until it caused a complication. Foot treatment, protection, and amputation prevention historically have been overlooked or covered only slightly in medical education. Chronic neuropathic complications have been seen to have an unavoidable outcome. In many areas, there are no certified orthotists or local health care practitioners who are trained in off-loading techniques. The goal of treatment of a neuropathic or dysvascular patient is to preserve the limb and ambulatory function. Techniques can be shared between disciplines for improved outcomes for neuropathic patients. The combined team expertise with state-of-the-art techniques have enabled wound healing, limb salvage, and improved quality of life for this high-risk population.

References

[1] Frykberg RG. The team approach in diabetic foot management. Adv Wound Care 1998;11:71–7.
[2] Blume PA, Novicki DC, et al. Skin grafts and flaps for the diabetic foot wounds. Biomechanics 1997;4:59–63.
[3] Jerrell M. Management of the diabetic foot. O & P Business News 2005;28–33.
[4] American Diabetes Association. Diabetes: maiming and killing millions. O & P Business World 1999;47–9.
[5] American Diabetes Association. Association updates diabetes facts and figures. Diabetes Forecast 1998;94.
[6] Nawoczenski DA, Birke JA. Management of the neuropathic foot in the elderly. Top Geriatr Rehabil 1992;7:36–48.
[7] Cailliet R. Foot and ankle pain. 2nd edition. Philadelphia: Davis; 1983.

[8] American Diabetes Association. Taming the pain of nerve disease. Diabetes Advisor 1999;14.

[9] Yale JF. Yale's podiatric medicine. 3rd edition. Baltimore: Williams & Wilkins; 1987.

[10] American Diabetes Association. Possible relief on the way for some nerve pain sufferers. Diabetes Forecast 1998;71.

[11] Berne RM, Levy MN. Physiology. St Louis: Mosby-Year Book; 1993. p. 244–59.

[12] Levin ME, O'Neal LW, et al. The diabetic foot. 5th edition. St Louis: Mosby-Year Book; 1993.

[13] Armstrong DG, Lavery LA. Diabetic classification—7 questions you should ask. Podiatry Today 1997;32–9.

[14] Sandrow RE, Toro JS, et al. The use of thermography in the early diagnosis of neuropathic arthropathy in the feet of diabetics. Clin Orthop 1972;88:31–3.

[15] Sussman C, Bates-Jensen BM. Wound care: a collaborative practice manual for physical therapists and nurses. Gaithersburg (MD): Aspen Publishers; 1998.

[16] Horsley NL. Detecting and managing limb length discrepancy. Podiatry Today 1996;54–61.

[17] Okun SJ, Morgan JW, et al. Limb length discrepancy, a new method of measurement and its clinical significance. J Am Podiatr Assoc 1982;72:595–9.

[18] Bowker JH. Identifying the limits of nonsurgical management of the diabetic foot problems. Biomechanics 1997;4:73–4.

[19] Armstrong DG, Lavery LA. Predicting neuropathic ulceration with infrared dermal thermography. J Am Podiatr Assoc 1997;87:336–7.

[20] Lavery L, Higgins K, Lanctot D, et al. Home monitoring of skin temperatures to prevent ulceration. Diabetes Care 2004;27:2642–7.

[21] Armstrong DG, Lavery LA, et al. Infrared dermal thermometry for the high-risk diabetic foot. Phys Ther 1997;77:169–77.

[22] Horzic M, Bunoza D, et al. Contact thermography in a study of primary healing of surgical wounds. Ostomy Wound Manage 1996;42:36–42.

[23] American Physical Rehabilitation Network. Functional locomotor biomechanical exam. Practical Program 1984;24–5.

[24] Davis AJ. Biomechanics and the diabetic boot: the University of Michigan experience. Proceedings 1996 AOPA National Assembly, Cincinnati (OH), October 29, 1996.

[25] Giacalone VF. Diabetic foot care: pressure-relief modalities. Podiatry Today 1998;16–20.

[26] American Diabetes Association. Diabetes-specific disorders: Diabetes Forecast 1991;1.

[27] Tremaine MD, Awad EM. The foot and ankle sourcebook. Carville (LA): Lowell House; 1995.

[28] Cavanagh PR, Young MJ, et al. Radiologic abnormalities in feet of patients with diabetic neuropathy. Diabetes Care 1994;17:201–9.

[29] Foster DB, Basserr RC. Neuropathic arthropathy (Charcot joint) associated with diabetic arthropathy. Arch Neural Psychiatry 1947;57:173–85.

[30] American Diabetes Association. Charcot's joint: are your feet at risk? Diabetes Advisor 1998;7.

[31] Grayson ML, Gibbons GW, et al. Probing to bone in infected pedal ulcers, a clinical sign of underlying osteomyelitis in diabetic patients. JAMA 1995;273:721–3.

[32] Travell JG, Simons D. Myofascial pain and dysfunction, the trigger point manual: the lower extremities, vol. 2. Baltimore: Williams & Wilkins; 1983.

[33] Sykes MT, Godsey JB. Vascular assessment and limb salvage. Podiatry Today 1998;32–65.

[34] Mulder GD, Jeter KF, et al. Clinician's pocket guide to chronic wound repair. Spartenburg (SC): Wound Healing Publications; 1991.

[35] Martin B. Blood flow determines capacity for healing. Biomechanics 1999;6:51–61.

[36] Fishman TD. Lower extremity edema: diagnostic strategies. Podiatry Today 1999;51–2.

[37] Heckman JD. Fractures—emergency care and complications. Clin Symp 1991;43:2–32.

[38] Armstrong DG, Lavery LA, et al. Healing the diabetic wound with pressure off-loading. Biomechanics 1997;4:67.

[39] Fleischli JG, Laughlin TJ. TCC remains the gold standard for off-loading plantar ulcers. Biomechanics 1998;51–2.

[40] Birke JA, Nawoczenski DA. Orthopedic walkers: effect on plantar pressures. Clin Prosthet Orthot 1998;12:74–80.

[41] Harkless LB, Quebedeaux-Farnham T. Total contact casting: why when and how to. Biomechanics 1995;81–3.

[42] Elftman N. The ODS splint. Biomechanics 1997;179–82.

[43] Ovington LG. Wound healing forecast looks wet. Biomechanics 1998;39–70.

[44] Pieper B, Templin T, et al. Wound prevalence, types and treatments in home care. Adv Wound Care 1999;12:117–26.

[45] National Institute on Aging. Age page—foot care. Bethesda (MD): National Institutes of Health, US Department of Health and Human Services, Public Health Service: 1994.

ELSEVIER
SAUNDERS

Phys Med Rehabil Clin N Am
17 (2006) 159–172

PHYSICAL MEDICINE
AND REHABILITATION
CLINICS OF
NORTH AMERICA

Robotic Orthoses for Body Weight–Supported Treadmill Training

Patricia Winchester, PhD, PT*, Ross Querry, PhD, PT

Department of Physical Therapy, The University of Texas Southwestern Medical Center,
5323 Harry Hines Boulevard, Dallas, TX 75390-8876, USA

In the past 2 decades, body weight–supported treadmill training (BWSTT) has been used to enhance locomotor function in individuals after a spinal cord injury (SCI), stroke, or other neurologic conditions [1,2]. This rehabilitative intervention involves supporting part of the patient's body weight over a motorized treadmill while therapists use manual facilitation techniques to produce stepping motions of the patient's legs [3]. Locomotor training using BWSTT is based on principles that promote the movement of limbs and trunk to generate sensory information consistent with locomotion to improve the potential for the recovery of walking after neurologic injury [4]. BWSTT is based on practicing a normal physiologic gait pattern, with attention to the ideal kinematic and temporal aspects of gait [5]. To replicate a normal gait pattern, two to three physical therapists are needed to conduct the task-specific training sessions to control or assist with trunk and limb kinematics (Fig. 1). Because close to normal gait speeds are needed to maintain the normal temporal aspects of locomotion, the training can be physically taxing.

The success of BWSTT in restoring overground locomotion has been documented in individuals after a SCI [3,5–8] or stroke [9,10]. Despite these reports, the use of BWSTT in most rehabilitation settings has been limited because of the strenuous and exhausting nature of the manual training for the therapists. As the therapists fatigue, it becomes increasingly difficult to maintain symmetry between the steps, an important sensorimotor cue used during BWSTT. Step-to-step consistency is hard to maintain. In

This work was supported by Grant No. R24 HD39629 from the Western Rehabilitation Research Network and the Mobility Foundation Center at The University of Texas Southwestern Medical Center.

* Corresponding author.

E-mail address: patricia.winchester@utsouthwestern.edu (P. Winchester).

1047-9651/06/$ - see front matter © 2006 Elsevier Inc. All rights reserved.
doi:10.1016/j.pmr.2005.10.008

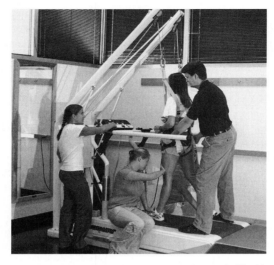

Fig. 1. Locomotor training using body weight support on the treadmill with manual assistance.

addition, most rehabilitative settings do not have the resources to commit the time of three individuals to the training of one patient.

Because of the drawbacks to manual locomotor training and to improve the delivery of BWSTT in the clinical setting, scientists and engineers are developing robotic devices that can assist gait rehabilitation. The goals are to reduce therapist physical demand and time, improve repeatability of step kinematics, and increase volume of locomotor training. Currently, three devices are available that are designed to guide the legs through preprogrammed physiologic gait patterns.

Lokomat Driven Gait Orthosis

The Lokomat Driven Gait Orthosis (DGO) developed by Hocoma (Hocomo AG, Florastrasse 47, 8008 Zurich, Switzerland) consists of a position-controlled robotic gait orthosis and the Lokolift body weight support system [11,12]. Position control refers to the robotic device controlling joint kinematics synchronized to ambulation speed. The Lokomat DGO has medical device approval in compliance with European directives on medical devices and is registered with the US Food and Drug Administration (FDA).

The Lokomat system is used in combination with a Woodway treadmill (Woodway GmbH, Steinackerstrasse 20, D-79576 Weil am Rhein, Germany). The patient is fitted with a weight-supporting harness that is placed around the hips and abdomen and fastened to fit snugly enough to minimize upward slipping of the harness when body weight suspension is applied. Primary weight support is through the outer pelvis and lower trunk, with additional support from attached leg straps. The patient in a wheelchair is wheeled up onto the treadmill via a ramp. The harness is attached to the ca-bles on the body weight support system. The patient is assisted to stand on the treadmill by the Lokolift body weight support system using a motor-driven winch capable of safely lifting completely dependent patients. The DGO apparatus is closed and secured behind the patient. The DGO is se-cured to the patient by straps across the pelvis and chest. Femoral and tibial length measurements are used to adjust the robotic force arm and robotic drive motor positions for the knee and ankle joints. Ankles are positioned in neutral dorsiflexion to assist in swing limb clearance with the use of spring-assisted elastic straps. When the patient is set up, the treadmill is started, and the subject is lowered to the treadmill. Treadmill speeds range from 1 to 3.2 km/h. The Lokomat DGO uses computer-controlled motors that are synchronized with the speed of the treadmill. Motorized actuators at both knees and hips are programmed to produce a normal physiologic gait pattern with attention to reproduce the normal kinematics of gait (Fig. 2).

The weight of the Lokomat DGO (21 kg) is supported by a gas spring that is mounted onto the swinging door by a parallelogram framework at-tached to the DGO. This design reduces the chance of the DGO slipping down on the patient. The parallelogram framework also maintains the DGO in a fixed position over the treadmill and prevents trailing movement induced by the moving treadmill belt. The parallelogram design and spring

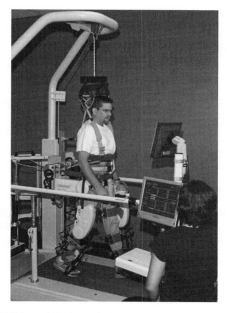

Fig. 2. The Lokomat DGO used during robotic assisted locomotor training with body weight support.

assist allow normal vertical movement of the patient during walking, but prevent lateral or anterior/posterior motion. The DGO has to control only the sagittal movement of the lower extremities.

Hip and knee joint angles are controlled in real time by software to achieve a physiologic gait pattern. Each of the four motor axes is controlled individually to correspond precisely to the desired joint angle trajectories. The drives at the knee and hip joints transmit assistive force through cuffs that are placed around the thigh, below the knee, and at the ankle and are strong enough to move the limbs even if muscle hypertonia is present, as is often the case with patients after SCI or stroke. To ensure safety, treadmill activation requires the use of either a handheld operator switch or optical light sensors. These sensors monitor the patient's feet on the treadmill surface throughout the training session; if the patient's foot drags, the treadmill stops immediately.

Adjustability

The DGO is adjustable to the anatomy of different patients. Several parameters can be varied to allow optimal fitting of the orthosis to the individual patient. The width of the hip orthosis can be adjusted for individual pelvic girth. The strap that is fixed around the chest of the patient is mounted to a back pad, which can be adjusted vertically and horizontally. The length of the thigh and the shank of the orthosis also can be changed. Finally, different sized cuffs are available to adapt to individual leg girth differences. The leg cuffs are connected to a right-angled tube that is fixed to the DGO. The tube can be adjusted in an anterior-posterior and a medial-lateral direction on the leg orthosis to allow alignment of the patient's anatomic axis to the joint axis of the DGO.

Body weight support system

The Lokolift is a dynamic, motor-driven body weight support system that allows constant support of the patient's body weight. Unweighting support is delivered through a single overhead attachment line that distributes the unweighting assistance equally bilaterally through attachments to the unweighting harness. An integrated force sensor monitors the precise body weight support during training. A fast response drive motor within the Lokolift integrates information from the force sensor and dynamically adjusts tension levels to maintain the prescribed level of weight assistance. The amount of weight support can be changed easily during the training session through the user interface. The maximum patient weight that can be supported safely is 135 kg.

User interface

The computer-controlled interface allows the therapist to operate the Lokomat system and adjust training parameters, including treadmill speed, the amount of body weight supported, and different gait parameters, without stopping the training (Fig. 3). Gait parameters that can be adjusted include hip flexion to increase step length, knee flexion at initial swing to ensure clearance of the swinging limb, and hip flexion offset to accommodate for individuals who may have a hip flexion contracture. Patient setup information and training parameters, such as hip and knee joint range of motion, are saved to the hard disc after every training session and can be recalled for subsequent training sessions.

An optional software module for the Lokomat system is the Guidance Force Control system, which provides the therapist with the ability to switch between position control mode (full robotic/DGO assist) and resistance free gait mode (ability to reduce the robotic DGO assistance) without having to stop the training. Reducing the amount of the robotic/DGO guidance force allows the patient to perform more of the movement actively and independently; this is particularly useful when working with patients after stroke. As opposed to position control, in which both legs of the patient are guided by the orthosis and moved by the drives of the Lokomat DGO according to the preprogrammed gait pattern, resistance-free control enables the patient to move one leg actively and to walk freely while the hemiparetic leg is still guided by the orthosis and moved by the drives.

Evaluation capabilities

The training time and distance walked are recorded for each session. The Assessment Module in the Lokomat system is an option that offers software programs to measure various patient movement characteristics by force transducers connected directly to the joint axis drives. The L-STIFF

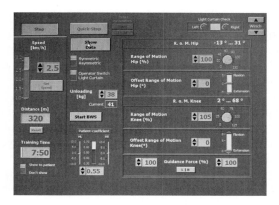

Fig. 3. The Lokomat DGO screen display showing the adjustable training parameters. Standard adjustable parameters include the treadmill speed and weight support. Lokomat specific gait parameters include hip/knee flexion range of motion, hip/knee offset angle, and guidance force adjustments.

software module measures the physiologic stiffness of the patient's hip and knee joints during passive movement of the hip and knee joints in three specific speeds: $30°/s$, $60°/s$, and $120°/s$. Results are given as torque values throughout the range or as the average torque. The L-FORCE software module measures the isometric force exerted by the patient for hip and knee flexion and extension while fitted in the DGO. Finally, the L-ROM software module records either passive (therapist driven) or active range of motion at the hip and knee.

Patient feedback

The optional Biofeedback System displays the patient's effort during therapy in real time on a flat panel display. Force transducers at each of the hip and knee joints measure the interaction between the patient and the Lokomat DGO during walking. This measurement allows direct feedback to the patient while walking, which enhances the patient's motivation to do as much work as possible and minimizes passive locomotor training.

Space requirements

The Lokomat system's dimensions are 400 cm long × 185 cm wide and 279 cm tall. The system requires a space of 550 × 350 cm with a ceiling height of at least 280 cm.

HealthSouth AutoAmbulator

The AutoAmbulator is another robotic device for BWSTT developed by HealthSouth (HealthSouth Corporation, One HealthSouth Parkway, Birmingham, AL 35243, USA), a commercial health care provider. In March 2002, the FDA granted HealthSouth permission to begin using the Auto-Ambulator, and it is currently available at 28 HealthSouth facilities. The AutoAmbulator consists of a belt-driven treadmill, an overhead lift, a pair of articulated arms, and two upright structures that house the computer controls and the body weight–unloading mechanism.

The patient is fitted with a hard-shelled harness that encloses the lower abdominal/trunk region with straps between the legs. Primary weight bearing is through the pubis and ischial tuberosities. The articulated arms are mounted to either side of the upright structure and are hinged outward to allow them to be swung out of the way when not in use for patient access (Fig. 4). The patient is wheeled up onto the treadmill via a ramp. The hard-shelled harness is attached to the overhead lift mechanism, which is capable for lifting dependent patients to a standing position on the treadmill. The articulated arms can be returned and locked into the operational position when the patient is safely supported. Each arm is designed with motor-driven pivotal joints at the hip and knee with links that are attached from

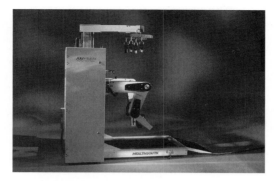

Fig. 4. The AutoAmbulator with the articulated arms swung away to show how the patient can be accessed easily when the AutoAmbulator is not in use. (Courtesy of HealthSouth, Birmingham, AL.)

the side at the ankle and above the knee of each leg using straps. There is no integrated attachment to control for ankle plantar flexion and dorsiflexion. Ankle position may be established using an ankle-foot orthosis or Ace bandages that therapists wrap to hold the patient's foot in neutral dorsiflexion as required for swing limb clearance. Trunk stability is provided by adjustable oblique braces that attach to the each side of the pelvic/trunk shell and to the frame to minimize pelvic rotation and ensure proper vertical alignment with the unweighting system. When the patient is set up, the treadmill is started, and the patient is lowered to the treadmill. Treadmill speeds range from 0 to 2.4 km/h. The gait drive components are computer controlled at the hip and knee through position, time, and distance to provide a normal gait pattern through variable treadmill speeds (Fig. 5). The AutoAmbulator is equipped with a light array to detect any improper foot placement. There are sensors at all potential over travel positions to ensure patient safety during training. In the event of failure, there are redundant hard stops that stop the training.

Adjustability

Proper height alignment of the drive mechanism is established by measuring from the ground to the knee joint. The arms are mechanically driven to allow the therapist to align the vertical axis of the knee joint motor drive to the patient's knee joint axis. Although the appropriate length of the lower robotic arm can be established in relation to the distance from the knee to the ground, the distance from the knee to the hip joint is not adjustable. This aspect may affect the robotic axis of rotation in relation to the hip joint axis of rotation. The cuff brackets allow the therapist to lock the position to prevent medial lateral movement of the legs during training or maintain an open position, which requires the patient to maintain lateral-medial stability. The oblique trunk braces may be removed to allow the patient increased

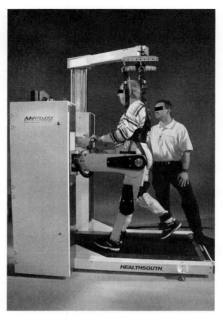

Fig. 5. The AutoAmbulator used during robotic assisted locomotor training with body weight support. (Courtesy of HealthSouth, Birmingham, AL.)

freedom of pelvic/trunk movement if desired. The AutoAmbulator allows adjustment of three discrete step lengths.

Body weight support system

The overhead lift is equipped with a rigid beam that terminates with a metal plate that attaches to the four points of the support harness. Force sensors located in the platform monitor the precise body weight support during training and report each side independently to the computer interface screen. The amount of weight assistance is provided through the computer interface and is adjustable during training. The weight support is static and does not allow vertical movement of the patient during walking. The lack of dynamic vertical movement affects the normal center of mass oscillatory movement during normal locomotion. The maximum patient weight that can be supported safely is 136 kg.

User interface

The AutoAmbulator requires minimal setup. Because the AutoAmbulator is currently only at HealthSouth facilities, the devices are connected to the HealthSouth network for diagnostics, upgrades, data collection, and service. The AutoAmbulator control user interface is through either a computer keyboard for complete control or a wireless remote, which allows for basic functions, such as treadmill speed and the amount of body weight supported. At this time, there is no capability to reduce the robotic assistance for encouraging patient participation or for a patient who develops improved active control during locomotor training.

Evaluation capabilities

Objective data include training time, number of steps taken, and distance walked for each session. Through the feedback mechanism, the therapist also can monitor the amount of force the patient is actively contributing during the step cycle.

Patient feedback

Force transducers at each of the hip and knee joints measure the interaction between the patient and the AutoAmbulator during walking. This measurement allows direct feedback to the patient during training. The computer displays the patient's effort during therapy in real time on a flat panel display. This display enhances the patient's motivation to contribute as much as possible during step training.

Space requirements

The AutoAmbulator dimensions are 236 cm long × 122 cm wide and 183 to 259 cm tall. The height range is due to the unweighting platform adjustability for patient height. The AutoAmbulator is compact and should fit easily within a standard 8-ft ceiling height.

Mechanized Gait Trainer II

The Mechanized Gait Trainer II (MGT) is another commercially available device with the primary function of assisting locomotor training with partial body weight support. The MGT is available through Reha-Stim (Reha-Stim, Kastanienallee 32, 14050 Berlin, Germany) and has Conformité Européene (CE) certification indicating conformity with mandatory European safety requirements.

The MGT does not work in conjunction with a treadmill, but is based on a crank and rocker gear system, providing limb motion similar to that of an elliptical trainer [13,14]. It consists of two footplates that are coupled to rockers. Two cranks provide the propulsive force. The crank propulsion has been modified by a planetary gear system to provide a swing-to-stance ratio similar to that during normal gait. Initial standing of the patient is completed outside of the device and is aided by the ability of the overhead support line and pulley assembly to swing out away from the machine. When the patient has the modified parachute harness secured, he or she is assisted to standing with a manually operated crank arm. When the patient is standing, the overhead support may swivel close. The patient must transition into the device, which requires ambulation with or without assistance into the device and turning around to place feet in the designated footplates. These requirements limit patients who may be placed safely and effectively in the MGT. During the elliptical arclike movement, the planetary gear system on the MGT is described as providing two phases of movement: a low backward movement corresponding to stance phase, which maintains a relatively foot flat position, and a forward movement initiated when the footplate is lifted 13 cm, traveling on an arc path returning to the initial foot flat position to correspond to the swing phase of gait. During the described swing phase, the foot is in an inclined position. Because the feet are affixed to the footplates continually, hip and knee joint motion occurs as a result of this closed kinematic action created by the elliptical path of the rocker assembly and planetary gear settings. The MGT controls the center of mass in horizontal (4 cm) and vertical (2 cm) directions by the use of ropes and cranks that are attached to the planetary gear system, assisting with weight shifting during training. The sinusoidal oscillations to control vertical center of mass are created by the vertical crank that is attached as the primary central suspension of the patient. Horizontal oscillations of the center of mass are controlled by a second crank attached to a rope that connects through the left side of the MGT and to the left side of the patient harness at the pelvic crest (Fig. 6).

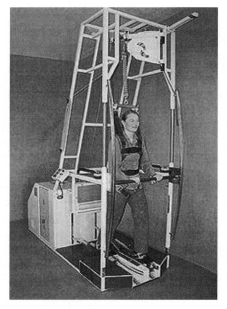

Fig. 6. The Mechanized Gait Trainer II produces an elliptical arclike closed kinetic motion that simulates stance and swing phases of gait. (Courtesy of Dr. Stefan Hesse, Free University Berlin and Reha-Stim, Berlin, Germany.)

Adjustability

Because the patient is not fitted to an orthotic device, there is no difficulty fitting the MGT to different patient sizes. There is a pediatric version that offers locomotor training for children with cerebral palsy. As stated previously, the MGT is most appropriate for rehabilitation of patients who have hemiparetic involvement or the ability to ambulate partially because of the requirements entering the device. Cadence can be adjusted continuously between 0 and 70 strides per minute. The MGT offers a stride length of 95 cm, but there is an optional variable step length from 34 to 48 cm. With a stride length of 95 cm, the speed of the training ranges from 0 to 4 km/h. Also, optional planetary gears are available that adjust swing stance ratios if desired. An induction drive servo-controlled motor compares the preselected velocity with the actual velocity of the gear system and adjusts as necessary. The MGT can provide full support when the patient is not actively participating, or it automatically adjusts the output when the patient either actively assists or resists the movement.

Body weight support system

A manually operated crank arm is used to support the patient's body weight. The static suspension coupled with the vertical center of mass variability results in the patient's perception of a normal physiologic oscillatory motion.

User interface

The user interface allows easy operation of the MGT, including speed, the number of steps taken, and the amount of body weight supported.

Evaluation capabilities

Objective data include training time and speed distance walked for each session.

Patient feedback

No specific patient feedback abilities have been identified with the MGT.

Space requirements

The MGT's dimensions are 255 cm long × 95 cm wide and 283 cm tall. A pediatric model is offered that lowers the overall height requirement.

Functional outcomes

Clinicians and their patients are most interested in the functional improvements that may occur with a given type of therapy. Several studies have shown that manual BWSTT can improve walking in patients after SCI [3,5–8] or stroke [9,10]. Because of the newness of the use of robotics in this area, however, only two of the devices have undergone testing with neurologically impaired subjects reported in peer-reviewed publications.

The first device to undergo a controlled clinical trial was the mechanized gait trainer. The mechanized gait trainer was used in a crossover design to train subacute stroke patients to walk [15]. The experimental group ($n = 15$) received 2 weeks of robotic gait training followed by 2 weeks of manual gait training and an additional 2 weeks of robotic gait training. The control group ($n = 15$) received conventional gait training for 2 weeks followed by 2 weeks of robotic gait training and another 2 weeks of manual gait training. Walking ability as measured by the Functional Ambulation Capacity improved in both groups. The median Functional Ambulation Capacity level was statistically higher in the experimental group, however, compared with the control group. The difference at 6-month follow-up was not significant. Training with the mechanized gait trainer was at least as effective as treadmill therapy with partial body weight support and required less input from the therapist.

Another commercially available device, the Lokomat DGO, has been shown in clinical trials to be effective in improving walking speed and endurance in patients with motor incomplete SCI. Wirz et al [16] studied 20 patients with chronic motor incomplete SCI after 8 weeks of robotic BWSTT using the Lokomat DGO. Significant improvements were noted in the patients' overground gait speed, distance walked during a timed 6-minute walk test, and performance during the Timed Up and Go test. Only 2 of the 20 subjects showed an improvement in their walking ability, however, as determined by Walking Index for Spinal Cord Injury II (WISCI II) scores. The WISCI II is an ordinal scale (0–20) that bases the ability of the individual to walk on three factors: use of physical assistance, orthoses, and walking aides [17,18]. The lack of improvement in walking ability observed in this multicenter trial may be due to the lack of sensitivity of the WISC II because all of the subjects showed increased gait speed and endurance.

The use of the Lokomat DGO does not seem to produce better results than manual BWSTT. Mosby et al [19] reported no change in walking ability or gait speed after 3 months of robotic BWSTT in four patients with chronic motor incomplete SCI who had undergone a previous 3-month trial of manual BWSTT. All four patients had improved in their ability to walk after 3 months of BWSTT. Although they maintained their walking ability and gait speed, there was no further improvement after robotic BWSTT.

Foreman et al [20] investigated if muscle activation pattern was the same in lower extremity muscles during manually assisted BWSTT and robotic BWSTT. These investigators showed on the electromyogram that the quadriceps and soleus muscles were activated during BWSTT on the Lokomat DGO device, and this activity was equivalent to the electromyogram activity observed during manual BWSTT. The anterior tibialis muscle was dampened during BWSTT in the Lokomat DGO compared with the electromyogram activity observed with manually assisted BWSTT. Foreman et al [20] speculated that the spring assist in the ankle mechanism inhibited the normal activity of the anterior tibialis muscle observed during swing limb advancement.

HealthSouth's AutoAmbulator is now available in 28 of their rehabilitation facilities. There are currently no published clinical trials for the AutoAmbulator. According to a HealthSouth representative (B. Adams, Birmingham, AL, personal communication, June 2005), current clinical investigations are under way.

Summary

BWSTT has become an accepted standard of care in gait rehabilitation methods. This type of locomotor training has many functional benefits, but the physical labor costs are considerable. To reduce therapist effort and improve the repeatability of locomotor training, three groups have developed commercially available robotic devices for assisted stepping. The purpose of these robotic devices is to augment locomotor rehabilitation by decreasing therapist manual assistance, increasing the amount of stepping practice, while decreasing therapist effort. Current clinical studies have yielded positive and promising results in locomotor rehabilitation in patients with neurologic impairments of stroke or SCI. The potential benefits from robotic technology are significant for clinical use and research. As further research is conducted, rehabilitation therapists and patient outcomes will be able to contribute to the development of current and future technologies.

References

[1] Barbeau H, Norman K, Fung J, Ladouceur M. Does neurorehabilitation play a role in the recovery of walking in neurological populations? Ann N Y Acad Sci 1998;860:377–92.
[2] Barbeau H, Fung J. The role of rehabilitation in the recovery of walking in the neurological population. Curr Opin Neurol 2001;14:735–40.
[3] Wernig A, Muller S, Nanassy A, Cagol E. Laufband therapy based on 'rules of spinal locomotion' is effective in spinal cord injured persons. Eur J Neurosci 1995;7:823–9.
[4] Harkema SJ. Neural plasticity after human spinal cord injury: application of locomotor training to the rehabilitation of walking. Neuroscientist 2001;7:455–68.
[5] Behrman AL, Harkema SJ. Locomotor training after human spinal cord injury: a series of case studies. Phys Ther 2000;80:688–700.
[6] Wernig A, Nanassy A, Muller S. Maintenance of locomotor abilities following Laufband (treadmill) therapy in para- and tetraplegic persons: follow-up studies. Spinal Cord 1998; 36:744–9.
[7] Gardner MB, Holden MK, Leikauskas JM, Richard RL. Partial body weight support with treadmill locomotion to improve gait after incomplete spinal cord injury: a single-subject experimental design. Phys Ther 1998;78:361–74.
[8] Protas EJ, Holmes SA, Qureshy H, et al. Supported treadmill ambulation training after spinal cord injury: a pilot study. Arch Phys Med Rehabil 2001;82:825–31.

[9] Visintin M, Barbeau H, Korner-Bitensky N, Mayo NE. A new approach to retrain gait in stroke patients through body weight support and treadmill stimulation. Stroke 1998;29: 1122–8.

[10] Sullivan KJ, Knowlton BJ, Dobkin BH. Step training with body weight support: effect of treadmill speed and practice paradigms on poststroke locomotor recovery. Arch Phys Med Rehabil 2002;83:683–91.

[11] Colombo G, Joerg M, Schreier R, Dietz V. Treadmill training of paraplegic patients using a robotic device. J Rehabil Res Dev 2000;37:693–700.

[12] Colombo G, Wirz M, Dietz V. Driven gait orthosis for improvement of locomotor training in paraplegic patients. Spinal Cord 2001;39:252–5.

[13] Hesse S, Uhlenbrock D. A mechanized gait trainer for restoration of gait. J Rehab Res Dev 2000;37:701–8.

[14] Hesse S, Uhlenbrock D, Werner C, Bardeleben A. A mechanized gait trainer for restoring gait in nonambulatory subjects. Arch Phys Med Rehabil 2000;81:1158–61.

[15] Werner C, Von Frankenberg S, Treig T, et al. Treadmill training with partial body weight support and an electromechanical gait trainer for restoration of gait in subacute stroke patients: a randomized crossover study. Stroke 2002;33:2895–901.

[16] Wirz M, Zemon DH, Rupp R. Effectiveness of automated locomotor training in patients with chronic incomplete spinal cord injury: a multicenter trial. Arch Phys Med Rehabil 2005;86:672–80.

[17] Ditunno JF Jr, Ditunno PL, Graziani V. Walking Index for Spinal Cord Injury (WISCI): an international multicenter validity and reliability study. Spinal Cord 2000;38:234–43.

[18] Ditunno PL, Ditunno JF Jr. Walking Index for Spinal Cord Injury (WISCI II): scale revision. Spinal Cord 2001;39:654–6.

[19] Mosby J, Foreman N, Tansey K, Winchester P. Robotic training in SCI subjects previously trained with manual body weight supported treadmill training. J Spinal Cord Med 2005;28: 160.

[20] Foreman N, Querry R, Williamson J, et al. The reliability and differences of EMG during robotic and manually assisted body weight supported treadmill training in spinal cord injured subjects. J Spinal Cord Med 2005;28:156.

ELSEVIER
SAUNDERS

Phys Med Rehabil Clin N Am
17 (2006) 173–180

PHYSICAL MEDICINE
AND REHABILITATION
CLINICS OF
NORTH AMERICA

Postoperative Management of Lower Extremity Amputations

Tim Goldberg, CP, LPO

ProsthetiCare Fort Worth, 1550 West Rosedale Street, Suite 100,
Fort Worth, TX 76104, USA

Postoperative management of the lower extremity amputation continues to evolve as a crucial first step in amputee rehabilitation. Although the major goals of early rehabilitation remain fairly constant, external forces continually pressure the rehabilitation team to complete these goals within shorter time frames. The atmosphere of rapid rehabilitation for amputees stresses return to normal function as quickly as possible. Early ambulation is the obvious goal for most new amputees.

Immediate postamputation concerns remain unchanged. Wound healing and edema control are the first steps to restoring function. In addition to the standard wound dressing, a compressive stump shrinker should be applied as soon as possible after surgery. Additionally, the application of a removable rigid dressing (RRD) has proved beneficial in protecting the surgical wound and in promoting wound healing. The protective environment of the rigid dressing minimizes trauma to the wound in case of a fall on the amputated limb and provides controlled compression to aid in the reduction of edema.

Rigid dressings historically have been used as an intricate part of an early weight-bearing device, the immediate postoperative prosthesis (IPOP). The traditional IPOP for transtibial amputation consists of a nonremovable plaster cast with an alignable, removable pylon and foot (Fig. 1). This technique was developed in the 1950s by Berlemont et al [1] and gained fairly wide acceptance during the next several decades. In 1979, Wu et al [2] introduced the RRD, which de-emphasized immediate ambulation, but did allow for early partial weight bearing. The RRD provided the protective qualities of an IPOP-type cast, but did not allow for bipedal ambulation (Fig. 2).

In recent years, various manufacturers have developed prefabricated postoperative prosthetic devices. Typically marketed as "adjustable

---

E-mail address: TGOLDBERG@sbcglobal.net

1047-9651/06/$ - see front matter © 2006 Elsevier Inc. All rights reserved.
doi:10.1016/j.pmr.2005.10.009

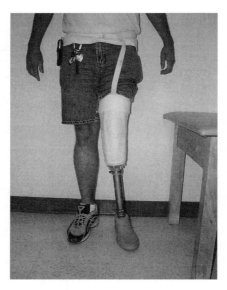

Fig. 1. Traditional plaster immediate postoperative prosthesis.

postop/preparatory" prostheses, these devices are modular by design and can be used with an assortment of foot or knee components. Consisting of an inner bivalved, adjustable socket and external frame, this device is relatively simple to fit (Figs. 3 and 4). Various iterations are available ranging from air-cast type sockets with removable knee immobilizers to transfemoral applications. These devices provide off-the-shelf expediency, but lack the intimate fit required for prolonged ambulation and for even compression.

The prefabricated IPOP provides a ready platform for early partial weight bearing, but is lacking in other areas. Because of the generic sizing

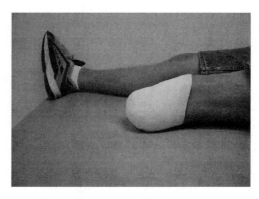

Fig. 2. Plaster removable rigid dressing.

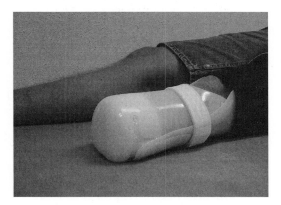

Fig. 3. Prefabricated plastic rigid dressing.

(S-M-L) and fitting techniques employed in their use, these devices by definition cannot provide an intimate custom socket fit. Uneven support of the residual limb occurs, and the risk for complications is increased. Excessive distal weight bearing and "bell clapping" or "hammocking" of the residual limb are common problems with poorly fitted IPOPs. Any of these conditions can compromise wound healing quickly.

More recent efforts have been made to combine a custom casting/fitting technique with the off-the-shelf IPOP technology to provide a low-cost, custom-made postoperative prosthesis. With input from Mark Bussell, MD, CPO (personal communication, 2002), a simple, effective hybrid has emerged. In January 2002, a 20-year-old man had a left transtibial amputation secondary to injuries sustained in an automobile accident. Three days postoperatively, it was decided to fit this patient with an IPOP. Because of his large body size, he could not be fitted with a conventional prefabricated device. Instead, he was fitted with a stump shrinker and a plaster

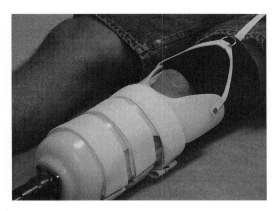

Fig. 4. Prefabricated immediate postoperative prosthesis.

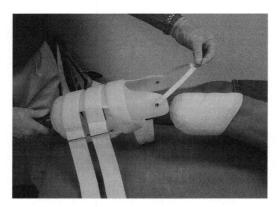

Fig. 5. Prefabricated frame with plaster removable rigid dressing.

RRD. Three days later, after significant reduction of edema in his residual limb, he was recasted. The external frame portion of a prefabricated IPOP with suspension belt, pylon, and foot was applied over the RRD (Fig. 5). The patient was able to toe-touch ambulate using a rolling walker immediately on donning the IPOP (Fig. 6). He continued early gait training with this device. One month and one cast change later, he was fitted with his standard preparatory prosthesis. Several other cases were treated in a similar manner, all with good results.

In 2003, it was determined that the original plaster RRD should be improved. Hygiene and ease of donning were areas specifically targeted for improvement. With the plaster rigid dressing, any blood or body fluids leaking into the cast could corrupt the sanitary environment. Also, the cast sock liner of the RRD created uncomfortable friction with the fit socks on the residual limb during donning. Finally, the symmetric shape of the RRD

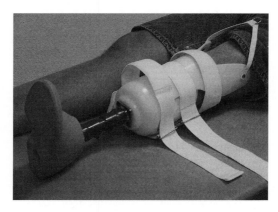

Fig. 6. Hybrid immediate postoperative prosthesis in place.

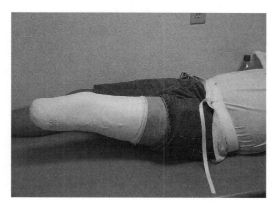

Fig. 7. Cast for custom plastic removable rigid dressing.

could cause confusion among caregivers, who often applied the rigid dressing backward.

Because most of the aforementioned problems related directly to the materials in the RRD, it was decided to replace the plaster cast with plastic. This change adds several steps to the process, but results in a product that is lighter, simpler to use, and more hygienic and provides positional support (knee extension). Instead of the plaster cast being applied directly and left in place over the patient's residual limb, a cast is made to approximately midthigh and removed immediately (Fig. 7). The cast is then taken to the prosthetics lab where it is converted to a positive model and smoothed. Heated polypropylene is vacuum formed over the model to create a plastic RRD. The proximal trim line is extended to midthigh with an anterior opening secured with an elastic/Velcro type of closure (Figs. 8 and 9).

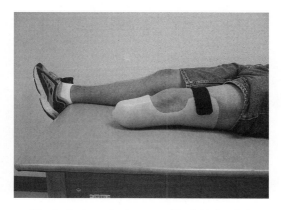

Fig. 8. Custom plastic removable rigid dressing.

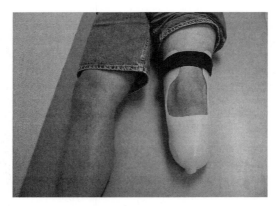

Fig. 9. Anterior view of removable rigid dressing.

This solid plastic **RRD** provides several inherent benefits over the plaster dressing. Because the plastic does not absorb body fluids, it can be sanitized easily when soiled. The high posterior brim and patellar cutout make positional orienting of the device obvious, and the smooth interior surface helps the device slide easily onto even bulbous residual limbs. A tighter fit is possible, enhancing compression and speeding reduction of edema.

After several successful fittings of the plastic **RRD**, the author proceeded to fit many IPOPs using the custom-molded plastic **RRD** in conjunction with the frame/pylon/foot of the prefabricated IPOP. This combination has provided what seems to be the best of both worlds in IPOP treatment: a quick, custom-made plastic rigid dressing/socket combined with off-the-shelf convenience and weight-bearing capability (Fig. 10).

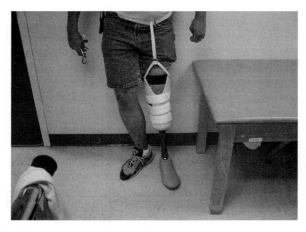

Fig. 10. Custom removable rigid dressing and prefabricated frame.

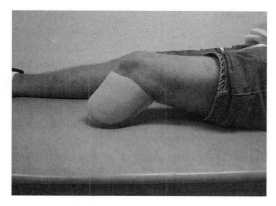

Fig. 11. Plastic removable rigid dressing trimmed for knee flexion contracture.

Another significant benefit of the custom plastic RRD is the prevention or treatment of knee flexion contractures. A common occurrence with trans-tibial amputation, knee flexion contracture often begins soon after surgery. The patient may spend the first several days postoperatively either lying supine with the knee flexed and propped on a pillow or side-lying with hips and knees flexed. Without stretching and range-of-motion therapy, this positioning can lead quickly to flexion contracture. Later, as the patient spends more time sitting upright in the wheelchair, an unsupported residual limb tends to remain in a flexed position.

When the thigh-high plastic rigid dressing is applied within 1 to 2 days postoperatively, these positional issues can be mitigated. Because the knee is held in extension by the rigid dressing, the patient may lie in the most comfortable position without regard to knee position. Because the residual limb is protected, the patient may feel more comfortable having it in a more

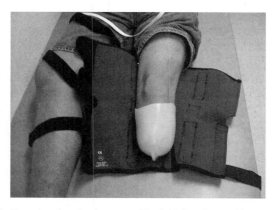

Fig. 12. Donning the plastic removable rigid dressing and knee orthosis.

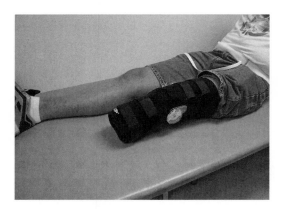

Fig. 13. Plastic removable rigid dressing with knee orthosis in place.

exposed position. Sitting in the wheelchair with rigid dressing in place and resting on the extended leg rest, the knee is again held in extension, while the residual limb is less vulnerable to accidental bumping.

The plastic rigid dressing also can be used to treat an existing knee flexion contracture. The rigid dressing is trimmed posteriorly to allow ranging of the knee joint (Fig. 11). It is then used in conjunction with a dynamic or adjustable knee orthosis to maintain constant extension force (Fig. 12). The intimate fit of the rigid dressing to the residual limb allows for the maximum extension force tolerated by the patient without creating undue stress of the surgical wound (Fig. 13). Further study is required to quantify outcomes regarding length of hospitalization and rehabilitation time frames, but anecdotal evidence suggests that IPOP treatment combined with aggressive physical therapy is an effective combination for early independent ambulation for new amputees.

References

[1] Berlemont M, Weber R, Williot JP. Ten years of experience with the immediate application of prosthetic devices to amputees of the lower extremities on the operating table. Prosthet Int 1969;3:8.
[2] Wu Y, Keagy RD, Krick HJ, et al. An innovative removable rigid dressing technique for below-the-knee amputation. J Bone Joint Surg 1979;61:724–9.

PHYSICAL MEDICINE
AND REHABILITATION
CLINICS OF
NORTH AMERICA

ELSEVIER
SAUNDERS

Phys Med Rehabil Clin N Am
17 (2006) 181–202

Triplanar Control Dynamic Response Orthoses Based on New Concepts in Lower Limb Orthotics

Marmaduke D. R. Loke, CPO

*DynamicBracingSolutions, Inc., 7798 Starling Drive, Suite 300,
San Diego, CA 92123, USA*

A new era of lower limb orthotics has arrived. Triplanar control dynamic response orthoses (Fig. 1) based on new concepts in lower limb orthotics are emulating outcomes found by amputees. Walking and even running with a natural gait appearance is now possible with triplanar control dynamic response orthoses [1]. Outcomes similar to what amputees have encountered in past decades are now being realized for some brace wearers. Preventing deformities and remodeling deformities that were thought to be fixed are possible with a variation of these ambulatory orthoses. Documented cases show improvement in velocity, stance-to-swing ratios, symmetry, sustainable velocity, alignment with angular improvements in three dimensions, less dependence on assistive devices, balance, function, duration, and hands-free standing. Other common benefits include less fatigue, decrease in pain, prevention of many surgeries, and decrease in falls.

The physician is responsible for prescribing the medical treatment plan. In rehabilitation, the goals are to help an individual return as close to normalcy as possible. The team the physician works with is crucial to success. The team focus is based on quantifiable outcomes for the individual in need. Each team member, including the patient, is important. The new orthotics technologies play an even more important role in enabling mobility as prosthetics have done for amputees. By definition, an orthosis [2] must accomplish all of the following: (1) support or immobilize a body part, (2) correct or prevent deformity, and (3) assist or restore function. All elements require forces by mechanical means. The ideal orthosis incorporates all elements stated in the definition.

E-mail address: MarmadukeL@aol.com

1047-9651/06/$ - see front matter © 2006 Elsevier Inc. All rights reserved.
doi:10.1016/j.pmr.2005.11.003

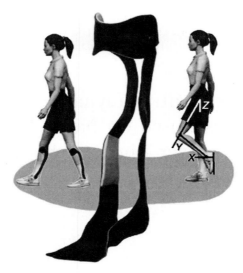

Fig. 1. Parallel strut.

There is new hope for lower limb brace wearers as the secrets for better outcomes by definition have been unraveled. The solutions for orthotics are more complex than the solutions for prosthetics, yet many answers can be found in prosthetic applications. The new bracing concepts [3] are governed by solving structural and functional problems by mechanical means to enhance efficiency. Underlying issues are addressed, such as security and trust while allowing forward, yet controlled mobility. Many new orthotics concepts are borrowed from prosthetics. Optimizing balance and dynamic balance with improved mechanics is planned in great detail. The new solution development incorporates a multitude of problem solving at every millisecond of the gait cycle in three dimensions. The underlying goal is to get all the body segments to move in the correct direction at the right time to obtain a symmetric, sustainable velocity to achieve efficiency. An adverse force causes a body segment to move in the wrong direction at the wrong time. Each adverse force ultimately detracts from the net force. All forces are mechanical in nature; learning how to solve the adverse forces and harness others for mechanical advantage are the driving forces behind the new bracing concepts. The new concepts are solution based with planned measurable outcomes.

Value

No individual wants to wear an orthosis or a prosthesis except when the device re-establishes balance and replaces lost function. This is similar to wearing eyeglasses. If the improper lenses are provided and an improvement is not noticed, the likelihood of success is slim. Individuals in need wear a device if they recognize its value.

The value of walking is often taken for granted by individuals not limited by physical limitations. Walking is the most popular form of exercise in the United States. The average individual takes between 8000 and 10,000 steps a day, according to the American Podiatric Medical Association, Inc; that equates to 2.9 to 3.65 million steps a year [4].

The value of a walking solution should be based on what it does for an individual and potentially enables. The value of the rehabilitation team should be based on outcomes they have accomplished in the past and the ability to improve outcomes for others in the future. With the new orthotics technologies combined with better movement strategies, many individuals can improve their quality of life while reducing long-term health and medical costs.

Complete or partial paralysis of extremities caused the highest number of restricted-activity days per condition reported, 56.2 days per year. The selected chronic conditions reported to cause the most restricted-activity days were arthritis (534 million days per year) and deformities or orthopedic impairments (469 million days) [5].

Rehabilitation is built on hope. Psychologically, an amputee would not be happy if an assortment of used or prefabricated prostheses were tried on them. Even if one fit well enough to walk with, the poor biofeedback the amputee may receive may set him or her up for loss of hope. This is no different for an individual in need of bracing. The individual may see no or very little value in someone else's used orthosis or prefabricated orthosis. Maintaining hope for meaningful walking is important to prolong motivation of the individual in need of rehabilitation. An orthosis should be designed to meet the specific needs of the individual, just as a prosthesis is designed specifically for an amputee.

Functional activities thought to be lost forever are being reclaimed by properly using triplanar control dynamic response orthoses (Fig. 2). The underlying key to success is better balance and efficiency. Understanding how to obtain these goals is crucial to the outcome. Returning function and efficiency to normalcy for an individual with physical limitations always has been the primary underlying goal for ambulatory lower limb orthotics. New insight and greater understanding has driven new solution-based orthotic concepts leading to better outcomes. New bracing designs have been developed by a culmination of factors to obtain better function and ambulatory efficiency.

Measurable outcomes

Measurable outcomes and consumer demand are expected to influence rehabilitation specialists to adopt the new concepts and put them into practice with positive results. Facilities with proven outcomes have the advantage in the marketplace. With the Internet, the patient, family, and friends are more informed and seek better solutions.

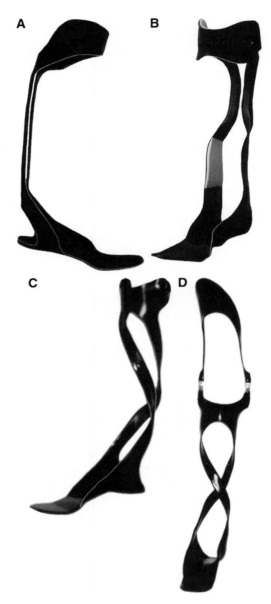

Fig. 2. (*A–D*) Triplanar control dynamic response orthoses.

The new orthotic solution development for balanced standing and ambulation is complex. The solution development is more than making an orthosis. Planning for dynamic balancing throughout the gait cycle combined with efficient movement patterning of the individual is involved, yet required to obtain outcomes similar to what is standard in prosthetics. Each individual and limb has unique requirements to solve. A solution for each structural and functional deficit at the appropriate time in the gait sequence and the appropriate movement strategy to work in unison is key to success.

Gait training without the proper orthosis offers limited value to an individual in need, as does gait training not taking advantage of the planned mechanics in an orthosis. Solution development is guided by many factors that combine a multitude of strategies. The process is much more involved than what is currently used in conventional bracing and gait training. The new solution development is planning for the new opportunities for each individual, after the data are collected and analyzed. The team must understand what is possible and design a movement strategy that includes the orthosis. To enable the potential outcome to be realized, the team must understand the mechanics and the process to support the individual's success.

The best solutions involve more customization, not less. Prefabricated orthoses and limited gait training have a negative impact on outcomes, rather than enhancing them. Although there may be short-term savings realized, the long-term costs for an individual who is not rehabilitated to his or her full potential is staggering.

Falls are the leading external causes of medically attended injury episodes (7.1 million episodes in 2002) [6]. Many falls can be prevented with better bracing and movement patterns designed to work together. Better balance and more efficient movement patterns translate into more standing and walking activities. Weight loss is a common benefit found in individuals wearing triplanar control dynamic response orthoses as a result of increased activity.

Underlying issues

Understanding the underlying issues that must be solved, the design elements, materials, retraining muscle patterning, and how they all should work in concert enables an individual with physical limitations to return as close to normalcy as possible. Without understanding a problem, a solution cannot be developed. Jonas Salk had to understand thoroughly the process of how the poliovirus entered the body, how it entered the bloodstream, and how it attacked the nerve cells that created paralysis in millions of individuals before he could develop a solution to neutralize the virus.

Physical limitations are most often caused by some form of neuromuscular or musculoskeletal disorder. Understanding each pathology, understanding their usual effects on structural and functional capabilities in an individual, and analyzing the unique aberrations for each individual are crucial. Designing a solution must take into account the future of the individual in need. Is there a progressive nature to the disorder, a stabilized situation, or a scenario where there is an expected gain in strength and function?

Normal human locomotion appears simpler than it truly is, and pathomechanical gait is far more complex than can be addressed in current conventional bracing. Learning how to solve every structural and functional deficit throughout the gait cycle at the appropriate time and return symmetry by mechanical means would transform the orthoses of today into a new era of dreams come true for the individuals in need.

People with lower limb neuromuscular and physical limitations are not only affected in the lower limbs. Most often, the upper extremities are at risk of repetitive trauma syndrome, especially in long-term conditions. When lower limb orthoses do not provide the proper structural control for static and dynamic balance, an individual is forced to use the upper extremities for assistance. The risk is greater if upper extremities are used to carry a percentage of the body weight. The more weight the arms, hands, and shoulders must bear, the more likely the shoulders, wrists, hands, and thumbs will be traumatized. The upper extremities are not designed to tolerate weight bearing for extended periods. Loss of leg function does not mean the loss of independence, but the loss of upper extremity function forces individuals into dependence on others.

An estimated 7.4 million individuals in US households use assistive technology devices for mobility impairments, the most frequent reason for using an assistive device. Almost 5 million individuals use canes, the most used assistive device [7]. The more an individual with physical limitations must rely on assistive devices for balance and security, the more cognitive and physical energies are required to stand and ambulate. Secondary functional losses limit the individual even further, such as the ability to carry assorted objects, to walk with one's head up and be able to look around freely, and to carry on a normal conversation all at the same time. When the balance is affected, anxiety tends to increase as the ambulator negotiates the imperfect world, where easy obstacles of everyday life become great barriers. The new technologies in lower limb orthotics are decreasing the dependence on assistive devices, eliminating or decreasing the long-term stresses on hands, arms, and shoulder girdle. The new technologies are enabling many individuals to regain function thought to be lost forever.

The new lower limb concepts are supported by science. Evidence, quantification, data, and outcomes are showing these concepts have validity. The mechanical laws that govern orthotics are the same as the laws that govern prosthetics. Mechanical laws are measurable. What can be measured can be compared. Baselines must be established for each individual, and new data must be collected periodically. Knowing what to evaluate, what to measure, and how to do it with accuracy is important (Tables 1–3).

Case studies

Patient no. 1

A 45-year-old woman was in a car accident in 1989 that resulted in a T12 spinal cord injury. She had subsequent spinal surgery in 1990. She

Table 1
Patient characteristics

Patient	Gender	Age	Disability	Length of disability	Gait abnormalities
1	Female	45	SCI—incomplete	17 y	See below 1
2	Male	63	Postpolio	55 y	See below 2
3	Female	35	SCI—incomplete	11 y	See below 3
4	Female	49	CMT	22 y	See below 4
5	Male	42	CMT	17 y	See below 5

1. Left gait abnormalities:
   a. Stance:
      (1) Unstable knee (buckles in stance)
      (2) Unstable ankle (varus moment in stance)
      (3) Excessive contralateral trunk displacement
   b. Swing:
      (1) Drop foot
      (2) Excessive hip and knee flexion
2. Gait abnormalities:
   1. Stance:
      (b) Unstable knees (buckle in stance)
      (c) 37° left genu valgum, 17° right genu recurvatum
      (d) 12° left genu valgum, 13° right genu varum
      (e) Excessive bilateral contralateral trunk displacement
   2. Swing:
      (a) Left drop foot
      (b) Left circumduction
   3. Gait abnormalities: steppage gait, bilateral contralateral trunk displacement
   4. Gait abnormalities: steppage gait, genu recurvatum
   5. Gait abnormalities: steppage gait, bilateral contralateral trunk displacement

Abbreviation: SCI, spinal cord injury.
Data from DynamicBracingSolutions, Inc.

experienced 14 years of disability with a left limb that was largely flail. There is no below knee or knee joint function with the left quadriceps measuring a grade 1. In stance, the knee joint buckled. The trunk compensated with excessive contralateral displacement. In swing, there was left drop foot and excessive hip and knee flexion to compensate to clear the ground.

Table 2
Gait characteristics of five subjects

Patient	Velocity (ft/min)			Stride length (inches)			Endurance		
	w/o	Con.	DB	w/o	Con.	DB	w/o	Con.	DB
1	31.8	77.7	157	21	25.3	34.6	50 ft	1/2 mile	2 miles
2	68.1	45.7	111.5	30.9	21.29	35.69	100 ft	100 ft	500 ft
3	66.1	54.3	176.6	22.08	24.21	44.86	300 ft	1/2 mile	2 miles
4	157.3	178.6	231.1	38.7	41.8	47.6	1/2 mile	1 mile	3 miles
5	102.2	118.6	138.1	28.1	32.6	35.7	300 ft	1000 ft	1 mile
Mean	*85.1*	*94.98*	*162.9*	*28.2*	*29*	*39.7*	*678 ft*	*1381 ft*	*8548 ft*

Abbreviations: Con, conventional bracing; DB, dynamic bracing solutions; w/o, barefoot.

Table 3
Stance-to-swing ratios

Patient	Left stance-to-swing ratio			Right stance-to-swing ratio		
	w/o	Con.	DB	w/o	Con.	DB
1	80.7:19.3	67.4:32.6	57.6:42.4	88:12	69.4:30.6	60.6:39.4
2	69.1:30.9	75.8:24.2	70.2:29.8	79.1:20.9	80:20	71.4:28.6
3	76.6:29.4	80.7:19.3	70:30	78:22	56.7:43.3	69.2:30.8
4	67.6:32.4	65.7:34.2	64.5:35.5	64.5:35.5	68.6:31.4	63.3:36.7
5	69.2:30.8	72.3:27.7	63.7:36.3	71:29	67.2:32.8	62.8:37.2

Abbreviations: Con, conventional bracing; DB, dynamic bracing solutions; w/o, barefoot.

There was a progression in functional development from walking barefoot, walking with a conventional orthosis, and walking with a dynamic response orthosis. All the measurements indicated a positive outcome: increase in the step length, stride length, stride duration, and walking speed. The stance-to-swing ratios also progressively improved from asymmetry to symmetry as they got closer to the normal biomechanical ratio of 60:40 (Fig. 3). The primary factors in increasing the walking speed were increasing the left and right step lengths and decreasing the stride duration. The symmetry of each limb to the other was another important factor in increasing the walking speed.

Patient no. 2

A 63-year-old man contracted polio at age 8 in 1951. He experienced 52 years of disability with a left limb that was largely flail and a right limb that

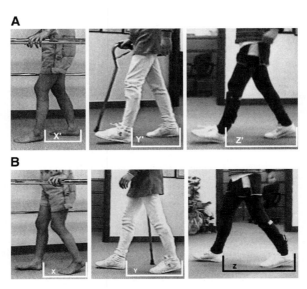

Fig. 3. Patient no. 1. (*A*) Left step length. (*B*) Right step length.

was normal below the knee, but that had nonfunctioning quadriceps and hamstrings. In stance, the left and right knee joints could buckle if there was any knee flexion. As a result, bilateral genu recurvatum had progressed to stabilize the knees. On the left in stance, there was 37° genu recurvatum and 12° genu valgum. On the left in swing, there was drop foot and circumduction. On the right in stance, there is 17° genu recurvatum, 13° genu varum, and excessive contralateral trunk displacement. The left limb in swing was functionally normal (Fig. 4).

Patient no. 3

A 35-year-old woman received a gunshot wound to the lower back 8 years ago. She was partially paralyzed below the waist and consequently was wheelchair bound for several years. Conventional polypropylene ankle-foot orthoses (AFOs) helped her to start ambulating a few years ago. The fitting of dynamic response AFOs made her independent and wheelchair-free (Fig. 5).

Patient no. 4

A 49-year-old woman had Charcot-Marie-Tooth disease (CMT) diagnosed 19 years ago and functioned well with conventional polypropylene AFOs with good endurance. The primary problem was a left genu recurvatum of 19° that could not be controlled with the conventional AFOs. She was fitted 2 years ago with dynamic response AFOs that controlled the recurvatum and increased the walking speed and endurance.

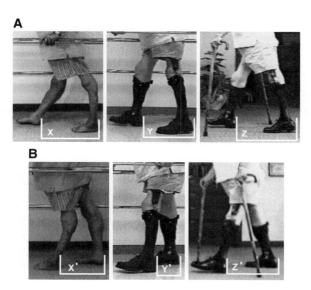

Fig. 4. Patient no. 2. (*A*) Right step length. (*B*) Left step length.

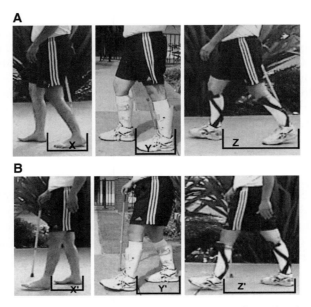

Fig. 5. Patient no. 3. (*A*) Right step length. (*B*) Left step length.

Patient no. 5

A 42-year-old man had CMT diagnosed 14 years ago. He had deformities of the feet and ankles, but could function with conventional AFOs. His walking speed and endurance increased with dynamic response AFOs, and the feet were corrected.

Discussion

One must understand the difference between biomechanics and pathomechanics. *Biomechanics* is the study of normal locomotion, whereas *pathomechanics* is biomechanics gone wrong. Biomechanics is very complex; gait laboratories around the world have developed an endless amount of documentation attempting to describe normalcy at every millisecond of the gait cycle. These laboratories have proved no two normal individuals are alike. Pathomechanics is unique to each individual and broken down even further by each limb. Gait studies show the disparities of pathologic gait patterns are greater even when studying similar pathologic problems compared with the normal population.

Pathomechanical conditions require more time and analysis in more depth than current practices of today. Studying videotapes of each individual in regular and slow motion, frame for frame, forward and backward with views from anterior-posterior and medial-lateral provides a tremendous amount of data. Every bony segmental deviation of the foot and up the skeletal chain in each plane must be analyzed to help solve the structural deficits. The functional deficits must be noted, and the analysis of compensatory movements is important to understand. Learning and understanding what causes each deficit helps guide how to solve the deficits at each aspect of the gait cycle.

The better one can assess the problem, realign the bony segments in each dimension, re-establish the mechanical levers, and replace lost function, the better an orthotist can enable an individual with physical limitations to achieve a greater potential. Understanding who is predisposed to pathomechanical changes is key to preventive care and minimizing the long-term rehabilitation required. An individual with normal biomechanics with neuromuscular deficits is much easier to rehabilitate than an individual with pathomechanical deficits compounding the neuromuscular deficits.

Pathomechanical changes start from the onset. Treatment depends on the severity of the condition. Range-of-motion and muscle strength baselines assist in determining preventive treatment options. Range of motion and flexibility are as important, if not more important, than muscle strength for efficient mobility in an individual with neuromuscular deficits. Contractures and ligament laxities limit efficient and secure mobility. The severity of contractures and ligament laxities dictates an individual's potential and dictates the complexity level of the bracing and walking solution.

A nondeformed limb is much easier to protect and control than a deformed and inflexible limb. The skin pressures between the brace and the limb also are reduced. The flexible limb with ligament and tendon laxities requires more corrective forces to realign the limb than a limb with all ligaments and tendons intact. The skin pressures increase as severity of the deformities and contractures increase in each plane.

Many fixed deformities can be improved by remodeling techniques. This remodeling requires experienced triplanar control techniques and unique bracing technologies along with advanced skills. Remodeling techniques have been used with success for various foot, ankle, and knee deformities. The principle behind remodeling is not new. It uses the same principles as orthodontists use for bracing and correcting teeth. Pressure over time can obtain impressive outcomes with no surgical side effects. Remodeling demands more time and understanding by the patient and supporting team.

Preventative measures

An orthotist who specializes in prevention of contracture development in all phases of rehabilitation is a great asset for the rehabilitation team, especially for the individuals in need of protection. It is important to initiate the prevention as early as possible before deformities start to develop [2]. If treatment starts after a deformity is recognized, the goal is to realign in three dimensions and prevent further predictable progression of the deformity.

An orthotist who specializes in prevention of ligament laxities is crucial for long-term care and efficient mobility. Ligament laxities are developed by unprotected stresses to ligaments and tendons under load-bearing conditions, such as standing and walking. Simple orthotic devices are ill equipped to prevent predictable deformities from developing. Any device that can be flexed or twisted by hand is not strong enough to protect the ligaments when protection is most needed under load-bearing conditions.

It is the author's belief that all ambulatory orthoses should incorporate triplanar control because ligaments and tendons are at predictable risk. A normally aligned limb with flaccid paralysis of a lower limb usually develops an internal rotary pattern (IRP), and upper motor neuron disruptions usually follow an external rotary pattern (ERP) [8]. Some upper motor neuron disorders show ERP in the swing phase and early stance phase, then break out of pattern into an IRP at midstance through terminal stance. Some neuromuscular conditions (ie, CMT, a genetic disorder that affects the nerves) create muscle imbalances. About 70% of CMT patients develop pes cavus foot deformities and follow an ERP, whereas 30% develop pes planus foot deformities, which follow an IRP. Even polio survivors exhibit both patterns. The better one can predict and understand the three-point pressure systems in the sagittal, coronal, and transverse planes to support, prevent, and maximize levers to improve balance in three dimensions, the better rehabilitation potential and long-term results.

The orthotist often is called on after all treatment options have been explored. It is common to see contractures, deformities, and ligament and tendon laxities already developing. This situation compromises everyone involved. The long-term medical costs are higher. The complexity level of care is higher. The probability of falls and dependency on assistive devices directly correlates.

The ultimate goal is to obtain efficiency. If efficient ambulation is achieved, all the underlying factors have been solved. An individual with physical limitations would like to walk from point A to point B with the least amount of energy. The ideal would be to return efficiency back to normal parameters if possible. The closer an individual returns to normal mechanics and efficiency, the more the underlying deficits have been solved.

Numerous good articles, chapters, and books have been written regarding traditional bracing in the past several decades. This article does not duplicate what already has been covered by these publications. Outcomes for conventional bracing systems have been restricted because of their inherent design limitations. Conventional bracing designs have not changed much for decades; the outcomes obtained by these systems have not improved.

Outcomes

Outcomes for individuals in need of bracing have not kept pace with outcomes gained by amputees. The advent of new space age materials did little for orthotic outcomes, while amputees' outcomes flourished. Why is this so? Why is an individual with sensation and partial paralysis of the foot and ankle, with good proprioception, quite possibly less capable than a transtibial amputee, who might be able to walk and run with an efficient natural gait appearance?

It is important to understand why orthotic outcomes have not kept pace with prosthetic outcomes before improvements can be made. Orthotics and prosthetics are governed by the same mechanical laws. Prosthetic designs and solutions have taken advantage of these laws to enhance outcomes. Traditional orthotic designs and solutions are limited in their ability to rival their prosthetic counterparts because the orthotic designs are often too simplified for the complex problems to be solved.

To obtain function for individuals in need of ambulatory orthoses, the mechanics must be solved. To solve many orthotic mechanical issues, one can ask: How are the same issues solved for amputees in prosthetic designs and solutions? Every prosthetic socket must control the limb in three planes for the amputee to position properly and to balance on a prosthesis. The socket also is aligned in three dimensions over the foot. Without triplanar control, an amputee would be limited in function.

Triplanar control

Triplanar control in orthotics is not new. Triplanar control has been used successfully in spinal orthotics for many decades, especially in the treatment of scoliosis and most total contact body jackets. Conventional lower limb braces do not implement triplanar control in their designs. In the late 1980s, Nielsen [9] introduced triplanar control to lower limb orthotics. Triplanar control for lower limb orthotics demands a greater understanding and time commitment from the orthotist to be successful. It not only requires the understanding of triplanar control of the lower limb, but also the developed skills and the application of these techniques to be successful.

To realign the foot, ankle, and knee of each limb is unique to the individual. To solve the puzzle requires meticulous analysis of videotapes from all views, frame for frame. One must inventory the bony segments in each plane and develop a solution to withstand load-bearing conditions to realign the weight-bearing column on which to balance.

Triplanar control in lower limb orthotics is complex, yet it is the basis of structural control required to obtain balance and security. The requirements of individuals with physical limitations who can benefit from orthotic treatment are no different than amputees' requirements for prosthetic devices. The better one can balance and be secure on a device, the better the potential outcome. The functional outcomes do not reach their potential until the structural outcome has been achieved (Fig. 6).

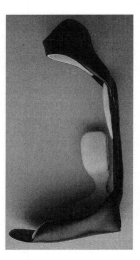

Fig. 6. Triplanar control dynamic response AFO with lateral phalange.

Triplanar control and dynamic response demand more rigid materials, such as graphite composites to withstand the stance control forces that normally would deform conventional thermoplastics. As with prosthetics, alignment is a key element to success. Alignment of a prosthesis balances segments one over another. Levers and weight lines are maximized to maintain the weight-bearing column in an upright position. Levers are important in the security of an individual. There must be a fine balance between enough security and allowing for efficient movement. A prosthetic foot can be aligned easily in all three planes to maximize the levers. With the orthotic patient, there may be fixed or limited deformities that limit the ideal alignment. It is imperative to maximize alignment for each individual for the safety of the individual.

Mechanical levers

Levers are crucial in mechanical applications. Although prosthetics have taken advantage of the mechanical benefits of levers for human locomotion, there are several examples of conventional orthoses not exploiting levers to enhance the outcomes for individuals in need. In prosthetics, there are no feet cut off at the metatarsal heads, there are no free dorsiflexion ankle joints, and there are no feet made from flexible thermoplastics. Everything that flexes in prosthetics is planned and has a controlled resistance. Most traditional braces cannot withstand the deforming forces in a planned and controlled fashion. Prosthetic outcomes did not excel until they used the resistance of the entire foot coupled with a dynamic response.

Stance-to-swing ratios

Stance-to-swing ratios of 60:40 (Fig. 7) are crucial for symmetric efficient human ambulation. Any imbalance of this ratio affects the symmetry, which affects gait efficiency. Symmetry is important for human locomotion. It enables energy from one step through momentum and inertia to help set up the next step in a fluid motion. The energy harnessed from this process is used in propelling the body forward, and when a sustainable velocity is maintained, human locomotion becomes very efficient. Any disruption to the dynamics of a symmetric, sustainable velocity has a direct impact on efficiency Any gait pattern that does not maintain a sustainable velocity continually must accelerate and brake a large portion of their mass on each step. The energy required to accelerate the mass on each step is taxing on the metabolic rate of an individual to the point that it cannot be maintained for long.

Pathomechanical gait

Pathomechanical gait patterns may have similarities based on etiologies. One may recognize a hemiparesis gait pattern of a cerebrovascular accident patient, a steppage gait of a Charcot-Marie-Tooth patient, or a gluteal lurch pattern of a polio survivor. When studied in great detail, no two individuals with a cerebrovascular accident are the same; no two individuals or limbs are the same with CMT, polio, spinal cord injuries, or any other neuromuscular or musculoskeletal disorders. The variable combinations of deficits seem endless and affect each limb and individual differently.

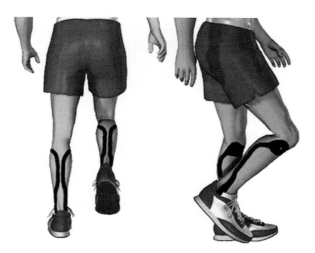

Fig. 7. A stance-to-swing ratio of 60:40.

Foot drop

There is no such thing as a "simple" drop foot. What appears to be the lack of active dorsiflexors is more complex and has consequences if not addressed. Understanding the origin, insertion, and functions of the dorsiflexors and their antagonistic plantar flexors and evertors provides predictable indicators. An individual with a simple drop foot develops a plantar flexion contracture with no opposing pull from the dorsiflexors or a natural stretch from a normal gait pattern. Without the normal muscle forces that support the longitudinal arch, coupled with a tightening Achilles tendon, a individual with a simple drop foot usually develops a pronated foot if it is caused by a flaccid paralysis. The midfoot starts breaking down; the calcaneus collapses into valgus. The 26 bones collapse in the foot following an IRP. Ligaments and tendons that link all the bones stretch or fail. All joints within the foot are triplanar in nature. The ligaments in each foot of each individual stretch or tear differently and at different rates. This is one of the reasons for unique pathomechanical conditions.

Levers, triplanar control, maximized alignment, stance control, and dynamic response are limited or nonexistent in traditional orthotic designs. Yet, these are the very concepts that have created excellent outcomes for amputees in recent decades.

It is imperative to realign each bony segment in each of the three dimensions to prevent uneven wear of joint surfaces. Muscles work at their maximum effectiveness when properly aligned. Balance and security are enhanced with each improvement (Fig. 8). Security issues must be solved before an individual can learn to trust a device. Security issues often are associated with falls or near-falls. A knee buckling anteriorly, ankle rolling over, or tripping over a drop foot are a few examples.

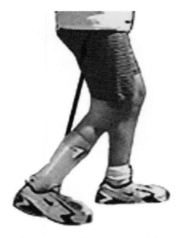

Fig. 8. Balance and security are at their maximum with proper muscle alignment.

Compensatory movements

Compensatory movements are soon learned to counter security issues. Compensatory measures for safety always sacrifice efficiency. Addressing the security issue helps reduce fatigue and anxiety and undo stresses on the structures required for the compensations. Designing solutions to address the underlying security issues solves the need to make compensatory movements. A prime example is the proper means of solving recurvatum. The security issue is an anterior knee control problem. The repetitive compensatory movements for safety have created the initial back knee until it develops into recurvatum. By using advanced orthotics floor reaction techniques similar to those used in prosthetics, the knee can be controlled, and with training, trust can be established to eliminate the need to pop the knee back on each step. By solving the security issue, the compensatory movements associated with the security issue are solved. Designing to solve the compensatory movements such as recurvatum without addressing the anterior knee control problem would lead to limited success or failure (Fig. 9).

Compensations are a sign of underlying problems. They usually are caused by security issues, balance problems, or functional deficits. Analyzing the cause of each compensatory movement in each plane and in each phase of the gait cycle is imperative. Compensations that use vertical strategies must be solved first because these are the most taxing on human locomotion. The vertical compensations are fighting gravity the most, magnified by the amount of the mass being moved. The next most important compensations to address are those in which the body parts are moving 180° to the intended direction of movement, such as recurvatum. Next in importance are compensations that are lateral, or 90° to the line of progression, such as a truncal lean or a circumducting leg. Compensations may overlap each other and form signature walking patterns. Arm movements for balance are common compensations. Some of the most common compensations, such as the toe grasp reflex and subtle arm or trunk movements, are not noticeable. Some individuals have worked hard to disguise their compensatory movements. Polio survivors were raised in an era when they were told to act normal and disguise their physical limitations. Franklin Delano Roosevelt fooled a nation to get to and stay in the White House. Every public appearance by Roosevelt was well choreographed, and ambulation was limited to just a few steps whenever possible.

Compensations are inherently learned for safety. They are good strategies until better walking solutions are developed. All compensations rob the individual of energy and symmetry. They all act as a braking mechanism while walking. This braking mechanism in turn must be replaced with an acceleration phase. Each compensation requires a measure of energy based on the amount of body mass being moved and its direction, plus the amount of energy to accelerate the body forward for each step. What may appear to be a simple compensation can require a great deal of energy.

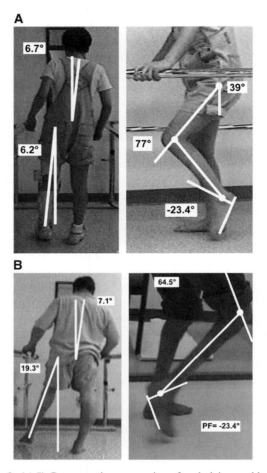

Fig. 9. (A,B) Compensations are a sign of underlying problems.

Compensations are made even with orthoses that do not offer proper control. Similar to prosthetics, if the anterior toe lever arm is too short, one may notice an early dropoff, knee wobble, or buckle. The amputee or brace user learns to compensate within a step or two for safety. If the amputee learns not to trust a device, he or she finds a strategy to get by. If the materials are too flexible to hold the body weight throughout the gait cycle, compensations are made. Triplanar control attempts to re-establish the natural weight line through the center of the foot to maximize the mechanical levers. If this is accomplished, and with a rigid enough material to support the limb, with training and practice trust can be established. The orthosis must be designed also to allow for natural gait patterns to be practiced.

The "clinic walk" can fool many busy clinicians. Most patients walk their best when they know their gait is being analyzed. Knowing how long it takes until they are fatigued and how they walk when they are fatigued provides more important information for solution development. Bipedal locomotion of humans is amazing. All the joints axes are aligned in such a configuration one wonders how it is possible to walk with no joint axis 90° to the direction of forward progression. Few muscles that have a pure single plane pull. The feet, which are the foundation, comprise 26 bones that can move in all three dimensions. The mechanical levers are very small from side to side, and the distal surface of the calcaneus is like a ball. The posterior lever of the foot is short, whereas the anterior lever is long. The knee joint rolls, then glides on a moving axis. The hip joints are offset ball-and-socket joints. On top of the pelvis there is a stack of flexible vertebral discs that supports the head, which approximates the weight of a bowling ball. What appears to be an engineering mess is amazing when every structure works in concert.

Mechanical laws

Gravity and floor reaction are natural mechanical laws with causes and effects. These forces can work for and against human locomotion. Learning how to harness their mechanical advantages and minimize their disadvantages is key to efficiency. Although the field of prosthetics has done an excellent job, the field of orthotics has lagged in sophistication. Because the mechanical laws are the same for orthotics and prosthetics, orthotists need to learn from the prosthetic applications of the laws to solve the present shortcomings with traditional lower limb orthoses. The clinic team also must understand how these mechanical laws work and incorporate them into treatment plans.

Floor reaction principles, sometimes referred to as ground reaction forces, are crucial concepts to understand as they relate to orthotics and prosthetics. If a foot hits the ground, there is an equal and opposite force applied up the foot and leg. Floor reaction principles have been used in orthotics and prosthetics from the beginning. The effects of gravity and the imaginary dynamic weight lines on the human body, coupled with ground reaction forces, are mechanical in nature. Learning how to take advantage of them throughout the gait cycle can offer a balance of stability and mobility.

Balance

Balance offers security and trust. An individual with physical limitations usually has lost the ability to balance and trust the affected limb. Standing balance may be re-established, but trust of the device and limb must be learned from repetitive cycles with proper patterning. When trust has been established, movement strategies can be introduced and practiced with trusted weight loading. The individual being rehabilitated must learn to balance with the body and become less dependent on the arms. Dynamic balancing is the key to arm preservation and efficient movement.

Support systems

The lower limb is better padded posteriorly than anteriorly, especially below the knee. It is easier to place the support systems wherever there is more padding. This concept has remained the standard throughout bracing history. Understanding support systems and human locomotion would dispel this concept as the standard for efficient ambulation. Support systems are available all around in the world. Humans seek handrails, countertops, walls, door jams, or other individuals for added support. It is often a subconscious reaction to the surroundings to use these items for support.

An individual in need of support from an orthosis would seek the support system wherever it is placed. If the rigid support is placed behind the calf or thigh, an individual in need would be forced to seek support he or she may desperately need posteriorly. The forces are directed posteriorly, and the forces are directed 180° to the direction of forward locomotion. The weight line is too posterior and body position with the knee back is not correct to initiate an efficient and balanced step. The step length also is compromised.

Placement of the support systems is crucial to stability and mobility. Efficient human locomotion requires all the body segments to move in the right direction at the right time. Every deviation from this norm affects efficiency. Support systems are placed to allow for more efficient movement and provide adequate stability for controlled movement. To encourage anteriorly versus posteriorly directed forces, well-molded pretibial shells are coupled with full-length footplates similar to prosthetics. The support systems must offer enough stability and still allow for planned mobility. The planned balance of stability and mobility is different for each individual based on his or her unique requirements and geometry.

Stance and swing phase

Similar to a prosthesis, an orthosis must control in the stance phase to be trusted. The stance phase requires the mechanical levers maximized, planned forward movement at the correct time, and a dynamic response; this propels the limb forward without excess muscle involvement or compensations (Fig. 10). Similar to prosthetics, the stance phase controls the knee from buckling and eliminates the need for most locked knee joints. Many knee-ankle-foot orthosis wearers can be down graded to an AFO using triplanar control dynamic response orthoses, even with nonfunctional quadriceps.

Solutions

The clinical team must imagine and visualize three-dimensional internal structural anatomy in movement throughout the gait cycle to develop

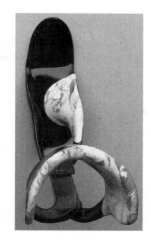

Fig. 10. Triplanar control dynamic response AFO with lateral phalange, top view.

walking solutions for pathologic conditions. Simple stick figures are great to describe what is happening at a given moment in one plane in simple terms, but they do not describe the complexities of the human body in motion, especially the foot. The better the team can visualize and solve three-dimensional deficits, the better potential outcome is possible.

Paradigm

Paradigm change is scary and threatening only to clinicians who are afraid of unsettling their current knowledge base. Professionals looking for better solutions for their patients do not fear the learning curve required to learn and master the techniques for triplanar control dynamic response orthoses. Individuals in need of orthoses embrace new treatment options if the evidence shows the options would help them improve their lives. The assessment process is more involved than what is normally required for conventional bracing and includes video analysis; structural inventory in each plane; functional deficit inventory; compensatory movement strategy analysis; stance-to-swing ratio analysis; range-of-motion and muscle testing; better understanding of etiology, pathomechanical conditions, and the individual's special requirements; and recognizing and understanding the uniqueness of each limb if bilaterally affected.

Rehabilitation specialists see patients much sooner than they did a decade ago. Patients often still are recovering from their acute stages. Acute care and rehabilitation clinicians must do a better job in the future to recognize and prevent range-of-motion loss and protect the ligaments when weight bearing is introduced. A patient's long-term potential is affected by even subtle changes.

Summary

With new insight and solution development backed with evidence, new medical tools for individuals in need of orthotic treatment are available. More research is needed to validate further and improve techniques and outcomes. More clinicians need to be trained and develop the skills to master the techniques. Outcome-driven results will keep raising the bar of quality and proficiency to enhance the lives of individuals who depend on orthotists.

Acknowledgments

Jean-Paul Nielsen's dedication to measurable outcomes and problem solving by mechanical means for individuals with physical limitations in orthotics and prosthetics will affect the profession and the individuals served forever. For the purpose of enhancing lives, he has pioneered several advances in lower limb orthotics and partial foot prostheses. It was a pleasure to have worked with him, learned from him, and codeveloped new concepts and technologies to enable and enhance lives. Mark Bussell, MD, CPO, inspired me when he went back to medical school to be the best he could be. He taught me not to be complacent with my present work. I have learned something from every client I have attempted to help. Inspiration for solutions often came from envisioning walking in their shoes.

References

[1] Loke MDR. Triplanar control dynamic response orthoses. Phys Med Rehabil Clin N Am 2000;11(3).
[2] Smith EM, Juvinall RC. Mechanics of orthotics. In: Redford JB, editor. Orthotics etcetera. 2nd edition. Baltimore: Williams & Wilkins; 1980. p. 22.
[3] Loke MDR, Nielsen J-P. DynamicBracingSolutions, Inc. Available at: http://www.dynamicbracingsolutions.net. Accessed February 14, 2006.
[4] American Podiatric Medical Association, Inc. 2005 fact sheets. Available at: http://www.apma.org. Accessed July 1, 2005.
[5] Centers for Disease Control and Prevention, National Center for Health Statistics. National health and nutrition examination survey. Available at: http://www.cdc.gov/nchs/nhanes.htm. Accessed July 1, 2005.
[6] Centers for Disease Control and Prevention. Summary health statistics for the US population: National health interview survey. Hyattsville (MD): Centers for Disease Control and Prevention, National Center for Health Statistics; 2002.
[7] Centers for Disease Control and Prevention, National Center for Health Statistics. National ambulatory medical care survey: 2003 summary. Available at: http://www.cdc.gov/nchs/data/ad/ad365.pdf. Accessed February 14, 2006.
[8] Redford JB. Principles of orthotic devices. In: Redford JB, editor. Orthotics etcetera. 2nd Edition. Baltimore (MD): Williams & Wilkins Company; 1986. p. 14.
[9] Nielsen J-P. Oregon orthotic systems; 1991.

ELSEVIER
SAUNDERS

Phys Med Rehabil Clin N Am
17 (2006) 203–243

PHYSICAL MEDICINE
AND REHABILITATION
CLINICS OF
NORTH AMERICA

Biomechanical Assessment and Treatment in Lower Extremity Prosthetics and Orthotics: A Clinical Perspective

Robert A. Bedotto, PT, CPO, CPI

OrthoTherapy LLC at Bray Orthotics and Prosthetics, 217 Old Hook Road, Westwood, NJ 07675, USA

Biomechanics is a term that is widely used by physicians, prosthetists, orthotists, and physical therapists to describe the mechanics of human locomotion. It is a subject that involves many fields of knowledge, including anatomy, kinesiology, neurophysiology, mechanics, physics, and mathematics. Volumes have been written on the subject, but even some experts admit, "Despite our fascination and years of scientific inquiry, we still do not know how we manage to get from point A to point B in an upright position. Controlling bipedal locomotion is not an easy task" [1].

The use of a prosthesis or an orthosis for locomotion adds an additional mechanical element to the study of biomechanics; as a result, the bio side of the equation representing the biomechanics of human locomotion interfaces with the mechanical side of the equation representing the prosthesis or orthosis. The sum of this equation is a complete biomechanical system represented by the patient; bio-mechanical treatment is required.

To provide comprehensive treatment, the prosthesis or orthosis must become an integral part of that treatment; however, as mechanical devices, they also are products. In this context, they have limited value. Although these devices are used in treatment, this does not automatically imply that they are truly a part of treatment. Treatment is a term most associated with physical therapy. The therapist provides physical treatment, whereas the prosthetist/orthotist provides the device. The mechanical device is a system composed of materials and technology. Design, fabrication, fit, and alignment also are part of the system, however, and these comprise a service

E-mail address: rabedotto@juno.com

1047-9651/06/$ - see front matter © 2006 Elsevier Inc. All rights reserved.
doi:10.1016/j.pmr.2005.10.007

provided by the prosthetist/orthotist, which constitutes mechanical treatment.

The goal of treatment related to prosthetics and orthotics is to ambulate in a safe and functional manner with the mechanical device. More importantly, how does the patient get from point A to point B? What is considered functional? Increased function is directly proportional to increased efficiency of the gait pattern. The efficiency of ambulation is increased as the parameters of gait approach normal; the ultimate goal of biomechanical treatment is to obtain maximum efficiency in ambulation. This goal requires the integration and coordination of the biomechanics of normal human locomotion, the physical status of the individual patient, and the mechanics of the prosthesis or orthosis. These complex subjects must be understood by physical therapists and prosthetist/orthotists and applied at the clinical level to achieve the desired outcome.

Previously in rehabilitation, time was not a factor. The duration of treatment was determined by a goal-oriented process. Preliminary treatment preceded the fitting of mechanical devices, and every case was treated individually. Prosthetic and orthotic management and training were part of the treatment plan, which coincided with hands-on physical therapy. The same team followed each patient throughout the rehabilitation process. On final discharge, routine follow-up visits were scheduled on a regular basis depending on need. A dilemma existed, however. Despite extensive treatment and follow-up, technology was limited; as a result, outcomes also were limited. The current dilemma, given the fact that technology has improved dramatically, is that time is now limited. Lacking is the integration and coordination of treatment necessary to realize the potential of modern technology. As in the past, outcomes will remain limited, unless clinicians devote the necessary time to the provision of total treatment. New advances in treatment must be introduced to coincide with the new advances in prosthetics and orthotics.

This article identifies biomechanical treatment protocols and methodology to establish a clinical basis for the interrelationship between physical therapy and orthotics and prosthetics. The information is offered as a compendium of the scientific basis of treatment and the essential elements involved. It is not the author's intention to elaborate on biomechanics, specific physical therapy treatment techniques, or orthotics and prosthetics technology; there are numerous references available on these subjects. The author hopes to stimulate critical thinking in biomechanical treatment to encourage a unified effort among rehabilitation specialists.

Rehabilitation treatment protocol

Times have changed, but the goals of rehabilitation have not. To rehabilitate is "to restore to a former capacity; to restore or bring to a condition of

health or useful and constructive activity" [2]. Specifically related to prosthetics and orthotics, the primary objective is to restore the ability to ambulate safely, efficiently, and functionally in addition to performing routine
activities of daily living. First, there must be a treatment plan. A traditional
rehabilitation plan includes the assessment, a prognosis for improvement,
and goal-oriented treatment. The need for a treatment plan remains as essential as in the past; it is more crucial today because of the many changes
that have occurred in the health care delivery system.

The delivery of health care services in today's managed care system does
not provide for a coordinated effort among specialties. Orthoses and prostheses often are delivered to patients before or after physical therapy treatment. In some cases, these devices are provided without any treatment or
input regarding the patient's individual needs or preparedness for the applied technology; as a result, the outcome depends solely on technology.
It also is common for patients to be treated in a variety of settings by
more than one clinician with varying degrees of expertise. The physical therapist and the orthotist/prosthetist may not communicate in a timely manner,
or they may not communicate at all. This situation results in different treatment approaches without a unified treatment plan. The continuity and focus
of treatment are lacking.

It is often assumed that the device provided will improve function. A
prosthetist/orthotist may fabricate a device that uses the latest technology,
but must rely on the physical therapist to treat and train the patient. A physical therapist who is unaware of the mechanical intricacies of modern prosthetic and orthotic technology is ill prepared to treat and train the patient
properly. The innovative and appropriate use of materials, components,
and design must be combined with the proper biomechanical treatment to
optimize function. The type of device and the timing of its delivery are based
on a complete biomechanical profile of each patient. Everyone presents
a unique profile; no two patients are exactly alike. Even patients with the
same pathologic condition have different profiles; treatment should not be
the same for everyone. Mechanical devices must meet the needs of the individual and function as biomechanical extensions of the body.

OrthoTherapy is the name selected by the author to define comprehensive
biomechanical treatment that integrates physical therapy and prosthetic and
orthotic technology. As a physical therapist and prosthetist/orthotist, the
author cannot separate the two. It is one treatment and is not separated
in time or location. This is not a new approach, but one that has been modified and simplified to maximize the potential of existing technology given
the present demands on time. It is based on the author's experience as a rehabilitation specialist over the past 35 years and remains a work in progress.

For a mechanical device to function optimally, it must become part of the
biomechanical system. The best description of biomechanics that the author
has encountered appears in the second edition of Orthotics Etcetera. After
an introduction regarding the purpose of orthotic intervention, the author

concludes, "Thus, the rational use of orthotic devices must be based on an understanding of how internal force systems are deranged and on the way external forces can be applied to correct the derangement. An orthosis must be viewed as combining with body parts to form a mechanical system that obeys mechanical laws and achieves mechanical effects" [3]. This also applies to prosthetic use.

OrthoTherapy coordinates the interplay between these internal and external forces. The physical status and mechanical needs of each patient are matched with the appropriate technology to increase efficiency and maximize function. This biotechnical matching takes into account the mechanical fact that the prosthetic/orthotic device also imposes external forces on the body; this is addressed in the treatment before and during ambulation. The body must be prepared physically and trained properly for the successful use of advanced technology.

The didactic information involved in a treatment approach that combines the bio and mechanical aspects of human locomotion, using a prosthesis or an orthosis, is extensive. To provide total treatment, this information must be reduced to its essential elements. Each element is then reduced to its lowest common denominator and applied at the clinical level. The elements involved are like the pieces of a jigsaw puzzle. The lowest common denominator describes each piece. There must be a clear vision of the completed picture and how one piece relates to another to become the whole; the whole can be understood by its elements. Technology and the scientific basis for treatment comprise the elements that make up the pieces of the puzzle.

It is easy for clinicians to become overwhelmed with information. The goal of OrthoTherapy is to reduce the various fields of knowledge into usable data that can be applied clinically to improve outcomes. Experts in a particular field of study concentrate on details. Given the complexity of human locomotion with a prosthesis or an orthosis, clinicians rely on many experts in all of the related fields of study. It is impossible to be an expert in everything; however, to achieve the best possible outcome, practicing clinicians must know something about everything. They cannot become mired in details. It is the clinical application that matters, rather than the knowledge itself. That being said, it is crucial to study the related fields of knowledge that pertain to human locomotion on a continual basis.

OrthoTherapy presents a different way to look at what physical therapists and prosthetists/orthotists already know, based on their education and experience. The key is to get together and learn from one another. Treatment that is based on biomechanical facts should eliminate opinions. The physician, physical therapist, prosthetist/orthotist, and patient must be in complete agreement regarding the treatment protocol. The OrthoTherapy treatment protocol follows the rehabilitation model with adaptations to ensure optimal outcomes. It includes assessment, development of the treatment plan, presentation and discussion of the plan (including short-term and long-term goals), commitment agreement, execution of the treatment plan, outcome, future plan, and follow-up.

In keeping with the puzzle analogy, one needs a clear vision of the whole picture before one starts. While treatment progresses forward, the thought process is the reverse. It is easier to see how the pieces fit together by deconstructing a completed puzzle. In this manner, the gait pattern can be deconstructed in terms of essential elements. Treatment consists of reconstructing the elements to produce the desired effect. Based on this analogy, one begins at the end of treatment.

Outcome

Optimal efficiency can be defined as being within the kinematic and kinetic parameters of normal gait. Kinetics involves the forces that control motion, whereas kinematics describes the type, amount, and direction of motion. Function is determined by the ability to ambulate efficiently in the community or workplace and perform all of the normal activities of daily living. Optimal function implies a level of efficiency, endurance, and safety that allows the patient to engage in a full day of activity given his or her age and health—whatever is considered normal for each individual. Goals would not be the same for everyone. Realistic goals must be set according to the lifestyle, health, and safety limitations of each patient.

A person's gait is like a signature. Often, someone can be identified by his or her gait before being recognized by sight. There is a wide range of normal. One also inherently knows when someone performs any activity efficiently. It appears effortless and automatic. A highly trained athlete makes his or her specialty look easy; however, it involves skilled voluntary movement patterns that have been learned over time and combined to form the activity. It is the result of repetition and practice. Walking is a learned activity that becomes automatic over time; however, habits develop with aging that identify one's signature gait. Often, the gait is not as efficient as it once was. If efficiency is to be restored or increased, the appropriate movement patterns must be re-established and practiced to become automatic. This involves motor learning.

Someone who walks efficiently is recognized by the characteristics of his or her gait. What is most noticeable is the posture or alignment. What combination of movement patterns is required to achieve this result, and how is it accomplished? An adult with a neuromuscular pathology or amputation also has an established gait pattern and level of efficiency that is premorbid. Technology would not change a preexisting gait pattern that is inefficient. This change can be accomplished only through treatment; technology works best in cases in which the individual has a preexisting gait pattern that is more efficient. Individual differences must be recognized that are still classified as normal. The same outcome, using the same technology, would require more treatment for individuals with less efficient premorbid gait patterns. Predicted outcomes must be based on the mechanical and physical profile of each patient and the pathology the profile presents.

The most simplistic description of efficient gait, from the clinician's point of view, implies that the center of gravity (COG) travels forward in the most linear manner possible at a sustainable velocity. It is implied that the vertical and horizontal deviations from midline are minimal (≤ 2 inches); the body is mechanically aligned and balanced; momentum (acceleration) maintains forward motion in a fluid manner. Inefficient gait implies that the COG travels excessively horizontally or vertically; the body is mechanically malaligned and unbalanced; momentum is not achieved because the COG may travel backward as motion varies in speed and direction. Postural changes in the form of deviations are the result of inefficient gait. Forward movement is offset by these conditions. The treatment plan calls for the development of a forward strategy.

The primary elements in achieving an efficient gait pattern involve posture (alignment) and balance. The body must be balanced in standing (statically) and in motion (dynamically). Physical and mechanical deficiencies are identified in the assessment. The requirements inherent in the appropriate posture to achieve static balance and the movement patterns required to achieve efficient gait are the focus of treatment.

Outcomes must be measurable to determine the efficiency of gait and the effectiveness of treatment. A qualitative (observational) gait analysis is a good tool for treatment, but lacks validity for determining outcomes. Clinicians know empirically when their patients improve. The patient looks and feels better. Regardless of the setting, there must be a simple way to validate and quantify the treatment. A kinetic gait analysis, measuring the forces that cause motion, requires the use of elaborate equipment beyond the availability of the average clinician. An individual functional ambulation profile can be obtained by comparing the patient's gait with the normal kinematic parameters of human locomotion. These parameters include velocity, stride and step lengths, swing-to-stance ratios, and symmetry of step lengths.

Velocity is perhaps the most overt sign of the efficiency of gait and depends on the other parameters. A short stride, increased stance time (reduced swing time), and asymmetry in step lengths decrease velocity. One author of a clinical study noted, "the best way to monitor the improvement of hemiplegics is to check the improvement of the walking speed" [4]. All of the kinematic parameters of gait involve distance and time.

The average stride length for adults is 4 ft, 5 inches—4 ft, 2 inches for women and 4 ft, 9 inches for men. The average range for cadence is 101 to 122 steps/min—117 steps/min for women and 111 steps/min for men. A slow cadence is 70 steps/min, and a fast cadence is 130 steps/min. Most individuals have a preset walking speed that is comfortable and normal for them and should be considered in treatment. Normal gait is 60% stance phase, 20% being double support, and 40% swing phase [5].

A baseline of information must be established during the assessment, which can be compared with the outcome. Many methods have been described to accomplish this task. The author has found most to be too cumbersome. The simplest, most economical solution requires a digital video camera, a stopwatch, and a homemade marker strip. Gait assessment without the use of a camcorder is laborious, time-consuming, and tiring for the patient. A detailed analysis can be completed with only several minutes of film because this can be reviewed many times in slow motion or one frame at a time after the patient leaves. There must be a sufficient distance (20 ft) for the patient to achieve free speed (the patient's normal speed). A lateral view of the patient is taken, walking in both directions so that the right and left sides of the body are toward the camera alternately. An anterior-posterior view also is used in the assessment, but the lateral view is sufficient to provide the linear measurements.

The marker strip can be made of any flexible material that is wide enough to make a legible "ruler" with bold indicators for feet and inches that can be viewed by the camera. It also is portable and can be used wherever there is enough space. It can be rolled up when not in use. The stopwatch can be used in real time while the patient is being filmed to determine velocity and cadence. Swing-to-stance ratios can be determined from a frame-by-frame review of the videotape. If the camcorder captures 30 frames/s, each frame represents 0.0334 second. In this way, the elapsed swing time and stance time on the left and right can be measured to a clinically accurate degree. Linear measurements can be taken from the tape in a frame-by-frame review by using the marker strip to measure the distance between the points of contact for the left and right heels.

This method is not intended to provide information for clinical study, but rather as a simple means to determine outcomes in clinical practice. It is intended to measure the relative difference in performance of an individual patient. The actual outcome can be compared with the intended outcome. The videotape also serves as documentation of the progress in gait and other activities of daily living.

So far, a simplistic view of the outcome and how to quantify the results has been presented. By looking backward, gait can be deconstructed into the component parts that affect posture and balance. By studying each piece and how it relates to the whole, clinicians have a better understanding of what to look for in the assessment that determines the essential elements of treatment. Treatment also includes the practical application of the scientific basis for human locomotion.

Kinesiology for clinicians

Ambulation and the implications for treatment

Clinicians deal with movement on a daily basis. Kinesiology is the foundation on which OrthoTherapy is based. Rehabilitation specialists (physicians, prosthetists/orthotists, and physical therapists) rely on kinesiology for the evaluation and treatment of amputees and individuals with musculoskeletal deficiencies. A clinical understanding of normal movement is a prerequisite for the assessment and treatment of pathomechanical deficiencies and abnormal gait.

Physical motion is the result of many factors, including anatomy, mechanics, neuroanatomy, physiology, posture, reflexes, sensory feedback, and subcortical and cortical control. For clinical purposes, the complexity of human locomotion needs to be reduced to the essential elements and understood in its simplest form. Ultimately, the clinician, not the expert, is responsible for treating pathomechanical deficiencies and improving function. Researchers devote their undivided attention to specific details and provide invaluable information; clinicians must use this input to treat the whole person in a timely manner.

This section summarizes the information needed to develop a treatment plan. It is presented primarily as an overview. The experienced clinician and the novice need to review the basics continuously and repeatedly throughout a career. Clinicians are not experts; they are practitioners. Clinicians seek knowledge and practice their skills so that they may improve the outcomes of their treatments. This is the only measure of a clinician's importance, success, and proficiency.

Kinesiology of normal posture

The evolution of the erect human posture separates humans from all other species. The postural changes from the quadruped position are the result of millions of years of transformations. There are inherent problems associated with an erect posture. Although the lower extremities have undergone drastic changes, the pelvis remains similar to that of a quadruped. The only adaptation in the spinal column is the formation of an S-shaped curve. Muscular development of the extensors of the trunk and hips increased, whereas trunk flexors have a tendency to deteriorate, causing internal organs to sag. This alters pelvic position and the COG, causing increased lordosis; as a result, low back pain is a common human problem. The upright posture also affects breathing and circulation in a negative manner compared with the quadruped position. Most importantly, balance becomes the most critical consideration in bipedal activities.

Although clinicians discuss static posture to describe standing, it is a relative term. All postures of the human body affected by gravity are dynamic. During static stance, ligaments of the foot can support the integrity of the bony structures only for short periods. Brief periods of muscle activity are needed to relieve tension in ligaments and prevent strain and collapse. There is a natural swaying of the body in stance. Although not obvious, it requires muscular activity and regulation. Standing is a balancing act in itself. Normal variations in posture affect standing balance to a greater or lesser degree.

Other factors affect posture, including visual, vestibular, and proprioceptive feedback from sensory receptors in addition to reflexes and reactions. Primitive and tonic reflexes are normally present during gestation or early infancy and become integrated by the central nervous system at an early age. When integrated, they are not recognizable in their pure form. They remain as adaptive fragments of behavior and continue to affect normal motor control. They may be evident in an adult to varying degrees with fatigue or damage to the central nervous system. Spinal level or elemental reflexes cause an overt movement pattern, whereas brainstem reflexes bias the musculature and affect posture. They are referred to as tuning reflexes. The term reaction commonly refers to the reflexes that appear during infancy and remain throughout life.

The righting reflexes consist of five separate groups: (1) labyrinthine righting reflexes, (2) body righting reflexes acting on the head, (3) neck righting reflexes, (4) body righting reflexes acting on the body, and (5) optical righting reflexes. Higher level reactions include righting reactions, which maintain the head in the normal upright posture or maintain the head and trunk in the normal alignment; equilibrium reactions, which serve to maintain balance in response to alterations in the body's COG or base of support (BOS); and protective reactions, which serve to stabilize and support the body when the COG exceeds the BOS. It is important for the clinician to be aware of these reflexes and reactions as they relate to balance and the mechanics of posture. The mechanisms involved in posture establish a baseline for understanding normal human locomotion.

Kinesiology of normal locomotion

In the evolutionary process, the foot/ankle complex is the foundation on which bipedal ambulation is made possible. The foot is a complex structure that functions to support body weight and allow forward progression of the body. Its functions include base of support, shock absorption, rigid lever system, torque absorption, and adaptation to uneven terrain. The ankle modulates gait and affects the proximal musculature through coordinated concentric, eccentric, and isometric muscular contractions in dorsiflexion and plantar flexion. In this context, the importance of the foot applies equally to orthotics and prosthetics because all mechanical systems are designed from the ground up. With the foot providing the foundation, normal ambulation can be divided into six components.

Forward inclination of the trunk

Forward inclination of the trunk is the movement of the body that initiates the first step. This movement places the COG closer to the line of force of the driving leg. Inertia is overcome, and the horizontal force of the driving leg is greater than the vertical component. Efficiency is lost without this movement because a higher vertical component causes wasted energy in hip compensations. All components must move forward. Trunk inclination increases with cadence.

Driving or supporting leg

As the trunk inclines forward, the driving leg propels the body forward as the ankle plantar flexes and the hip and knee extend. The second supporting phase begins when the swinging leg hits the ground. The vertical component of force of the leg supports the body weight, while the horizontal force acts as a braking mechanism. As the trunk continues its forward inclination, and the COG is directly over the point of support, there is a reduction in this braking force. Momentum is achieved.

Swing leg

On completion of the supporting phase, the leg is lifted up and swung forward to initiate another support phase. The leg begins in complete extension. The driving force of the hip and knee flexors initiates the movement. Dorsiflexion soon follows. This movement discounts the theory of the leg acting like a pendulum. When the foot has passed the upper body, the hip continues to flex, but the knee extends. This is not an active muscle extension of the knee, but a combination of hip extension at the end of swing phase, relaxation of knee flexors, and momentum.

Combination of swinging and supporting phases

As one leg supports the body and propels it forward, the other leg swings forward to contact the ground. In walking, swing phase never exceeds stance phase. An overlap occurs during double support 30% of the time. When the swing phase becomes greater than the support phase, there is a period when both feet are off the ground; this is running as opposed to walking.

The importance of the function of the pelvis in maintaining the ideal erect posture and its role in good body mechanics during gait cannot be overemphasized. The pelvis is one of the most important structural units of the body. It supports the body weight from above and transmits it to the legs. The pelvis acts as a universal joint between the upper and lower parts of the body. Pelvic motion is crucial to a smooth and efficient gait pattern.

Vertical movements of the pelvis

As the legs alternate between swing and stance, the pelvis is supported on one side, then the other, and both sides during double support. Velocity is key. The high and low points occur when the COG is directly over the point of support and just before the swing leg hits the ground.

Rotation of the pelvis

Although no component of gait can be singled out as being more important than any other, pelvic rotation is the mechanism that modulates and coordinates the walking pattern. It is the key to efficient gait. It directs the forces of the driving and supporting leg in the forward direction. As the swing leg advances, the pelvis rotates forward on the same side. A counter-rotation is required to keep the pelvis perpendicular to the line of progres-sion (LOP). Without this counterrotation, the thigh and foot would internally rotate, causing a serpentine pattern in the LOP, rather than a rel-atively straight line. The COG would increase its movement from side to side decreasing efficiency. The counterrotation of the pelvis on the opposite side maintains the external rotation of the thigh and toe out for proper bal-ance at heel-strike and early weight acceptance. As stance phase progresses, the supporting leg would internally rotate excessively causing toe-in and challenge balance, unless the pelvis rotates forward on the same side. It is easier to understand this mechanism when it is examined one leg at a time. During gait, the movements of the pelvis make it appear as though it is not moving.

Athletic trainers refer to this mechanism as hip roll. Hip roll improves ef-ficiency in fast walking and running by increasing stride (step lengths) and the duration of the force applied to the driving leg by the musculature and ground reaction forces (GRF). This mechanism should be understood thoroughly by the clinician and reviewed in gait analysis.

Movements of the head, shoulders, arms, and trunk

Humans walk with their entire bodies. The shoulders and pelvis act as a unit during gait. As the pelvis advances on one side, the opposite shoulder drops back to compensate for the pelvic rotation. The arms and legs form another unit as the arms swing in opposition to the legs. The arms serve to decrease the momentum created in the shoulders. By reducing the shoul-der swing, the arms indirectly keep the head facing forward in the LOP. The head has sufficient weight and without this mechanism, the head and neck rotators would be forced to work excessively hard.

The trunk serves as a torque absorber between the pelvis and the should-ers. As the pelvis and shoulders counterrotate, the trunk allows the opposing movement patterns. The trunk also serves to stabilize the long spinal column in all planes and supports the head and neck. The upper trunk works with the shoulders, while the lower trunk works with the pelvis. Trunk rotation should not be confused with pelvic counterrotation. The trunk absorbs the motion between the pelvis and shoulders rather than creating the motion [6].

This overview of the kinesiology of walking should be supported with a review of the required range of motion (ROM), moments of force created by the GRF, and the muscle groups responsible for movement or support at each joint during the phases of gait. These are components of the broader tasks of weight acceptance, stance limb progression, and swing limb advancement.

Kinesiology is the science of clinicians. Skilled motion is an integrated process involving many components. Ambulation involves automatic move-ment patterns that are cortically and subcortically controlled. A person learns how to walk. They cannot be taught how to walk. This fact has a major impact on treatment.

A human is a purposeful being. Cortical control separates humans from all other species. This cortical control allows humans to override automatic behavior even at the expense of efficiency. Ironically, the individual is not capable of understanding the nature of automatic movement patterns. Although it regulates all movement, the brain does not have the ability to understand the complexity and interrelationships of the many components of gait. Human locomotion is an unconscious and automatic activity.

How the body learns

Having assessed the components of normal gait, it is important to understand how such a skill has developed. Because ambulation is an unconscious activity, how does the body learn to walk? How do individual muscle groups form complex movement patterns? What is automatic, and what is within voluntary control?

In reviewing the many components of normal gait, one needs to look at child development. Reflexes and reactions combine with sensory input and feedback as the child matures. Primitive postures and activities such as rolling, sitting up, and crawling prepare the child for walking. Muscle groups that allow for these lower level activities develop into movement patterns required for ambulation. (This is the basis for treatment and gait preparation, which is discussed in more detail later.) Gait begins with a wide BOS, and balance is precarious. A toddler waddles side to side, and the trunk and pelvis act as a single unit. While the components of gait are developing, there is no coordination at this stage. Falls are common and frequent. As the child gains experience and confidence, gait becomes increasingly more efficient. Ultimately, there is no conscious effort on the part of the child to walk other than the desire to get from point A to point B. Input and sensory feedback from proprioceptive receptors, labyrinthine and righting reflexes, vision, and GRF combine to make adjustments in the gait pattern.

The central nervous system regulates this activity in the spinal cord, brainstem, midbrain, cerebellum, and cortex. After repeated and continuous effort, these mechanisms fine-tune the components of gait that eventually lead to an optimally efficient pattern of ambulation. The knowledge for this activity has been imprinted in the central nervous system through a specialized network of neural pathways. Humans take for granted the complexity of walking because they are programmed to do so. A child develops neural pathways from infancy that result in the skilled activity known as walking. The established neural patterns create a foundation on which to build. The human body is capable of amazing physical activities.

Highly skilled athletes take this ability to unprecedented levels. These individuals can react to new situations immediately and instinctively. They are able to build on their innate body knowledge and adjust to new situations automatically. They have an acute awareness of their bodies in space and rely on all senses to perform their amazing feats. The ability to perform complex and highly skilled activities efficiently and consistently is referred to as muscle memory. At this level, the only conscious thought is that of performing the entire movement pattern or the end result. The goal is a voluntary and conscious event. The performance of the activity is automatic and unconscious.

The neural pathways for automatic activities are imprinted in the brain at various levels; however, the cortex is not capable of understanding the mechanism of these activities or functions. The intellect of human beings can have detrimental side effects: Humans truly cannot think about walking and walk at the same time. Although the body can make automatic adjustments to unfamiliar or abnormal input, the cortex is capable of overriding these activities. In the case of uncorrected physical deficiencies, the normal parameters of gait are disrupted. Compensations for balance problems occur automatically; however, after a series of falls, fear and security issues become an overriding factor, and voluntary control of a part of the gait cycle takes over. Over time, these conscious or voluntary actions become automatic, and the new patterns become normal.

Motor learning can be defined as "a set of internal processes associated with practice or experience leading to relatively permanent changes in the capability for skilled behavior." Motor learning of new skills can be broken down into three phases [7].

Cognitive phase

During the initial cognitive phase of learning, the major task is to develop an overall understanding of the task or movement pattern. When the task is understood, the learner performs approximations of the task, discarding unsatisfactory attempts. This trial-and-error method of practice relies heavily on external stimuli, such as vision and verbal cues.

Associate phase

The intermediate associate phase of learning involves the refinement of motor skills through practice. As the patterns of movement become more coordinated with less error, the learner concentrates on how to do the movement, rather than what movement to do. Proprioceptive feedback becomes more important than visual or verbal cues.

Autonomous phase

The final autonomous phase of learning is characterized by automatic motor performance after considerable practice. There is minimal cognitive monitoring of the activity as the learner concentrates on the activity, rather than movement patterns. The movement can be performed consistently and repeatedly in various environments. Retention has been attained when the learner can repeat the activity over time after a period of no practice [8].

Assessment

Knowledge of the components of normal human gait serves as the foundation for treatment. How the body learns to perform skilled activities serves as a guide to treatment. The kinesiology of posture and ambulation serves as the direction of treatment. Finally, physical deficiencies and knowledge of pathomechanics and pathologic gait determine the focus of treatment.

The treatment plan is based on an assessment that identifies the physical and mechanical deficiencies and takes into account all of the elements of a prosthetic/orthotic system. Efficient treatment focuses on primary problems, rather than the treatment of symptoms. The mental process of deconstructing human gait, examining the parts, and reconstructing the parts to reach a goal leads to more effective treatment, including the most efficient use of time. Treatment is a goal-oriented rehabilitation process. It takes time and effort on the part of the physician, orthotist, physical therapist, and patient.

The assessment is divided into two parts. The first part is the videographic portion that determines the mechanical profile of the patient. This part of the assessment itemizes deformities, compensations, and balance issues that determine the specific need for external force systems (prosthesis/orthosis). The second part is the physical examination. Deficiencies and limitations are inventoried to create a physical profile of the function and status of the internal forces of the patient. The physical findings are related to the gait analysis to determine the treatment plan and the intended outcome. Depending on the timing of the assessment, the patient may not have a prosthesis or may not be able to ambulate without an orthosis. In these cases, the assessment would consist of a video of a postural evaluation only (standing and sitting), combined with the physical evaluation.

The objective of the assessment is to look at the individual as a complete biomechanical system. The outcome depends on the integration of the internal and external forces that create the whole system. It is important to limit the evaluation to the essential physical and mechanical elements. Many forms have been developed over the years; however, they tend to isolate and emphasize the details, which defeats the purpose of the evaluation. The clinician spends more time completing the forms than actually observing the gait. The most practical way to observe gait is to videotape the patient from the frontal and sagittal planes. In this way, the time required can be kept to a minimum, and the evaluation can be performed at a later time in much greater detail in slow motion or freeze frame.

Mechanical evaluation

Compensations or substitutions of movement patterns are the result of functional deficits to make adjustments for the deficit, maintain balance, and feel secure. In terms of mechanics, it is helpful to look at movement as body segment motion rather than joint motion. These segments combine to form lever systems that affect motion about a joint. Viewed in this way, prostheses and orthoses become external support systems that produce or limit motion of the segments necessary for appropriate movement patterns in gait. In pathomechanical gait, body segments show abnormal movement patterns caused by functional deficits and compensations. These can be broken down into layers as described by DynamicBracingSolutions.

The purpose of the mechanical evaluation is to create an inventory of all abnormal movement patterns at each phase of gait (for both sides). This information is related to the physical findings and forms the basis for the treatment plan.

1. The deformity layer: These are structural (skeletal) changes of the lower limbs including actual changes to the bony structure, ligamentous structure of the joints, and contractures. Movement in this layer increases with load bearing and progresses over time. Deformities are abnormal segment displacements beyond the normal anatomic ROM. They are the result of fusions or coalitions, ligament laxities, soft tissue contractures, and leg-length difference.
2. Neuromuscular functional deficit layer: These are segment displacements that are within the normal ROM for a particular joint, but excessive to the normal ROM required for ambulation. Functional deficits are determined by the individual pattern of muscle weakness, paralysis, or spasticity.
3. Balance compensation layer: This layer includes segment displacements that are within the normal ROM, but excessive to the normal range required for ambulation. These include trunk, arm, head, and pelvic motion necessary to balance over a lower limb misaligned by deformity.

The videographic information is reviewed repeatedly in slow motion and frame by frame to create an inventory of displacements, deviations, and compensations throughout the gait cycle. The abnormal displacements are listed for each phase of gait (left and right). These are categorized in terms of deviations or compensations. The observed movement patterns are triplanar in nature; all planes of motion must be considered for each phase in the assessment.

The segment deviations and displacements for each phase of gait are related to the physical findings in an effort to understand the abnormal forces acting on the body and the process necessary to counteract these forces. The physical deficiencies act as gait indicators and represent the internal forces that affect gait. Improvement or correction of these deficiencies combined with an appropriate external mechanical support system form the basis for the biomechanical treatment plan.

The postural evaluation relates the existing posture to a normal frontal and sagittal view of the skeleton. The ideal plumb line for a neutral posture connects the following landmarks: the earlobe, the center of the shoulder, the center of the hip, and slightly anterior to the lateral malleolus. From a frontal view, the eyes, shoulders, knees, and ankles should be horizontal. Displacements at the head and eyes, shoulders, hips, knees, and ankles are compared with normal. Balance should be assessed not only mechanically, but also from a labyrinthine and visual point of view.

Pathologic gait and pathomechanics

Pathologic gait is the result of musculoskeletal deficiencies and is characterized by various deviations from the norm causing inefficiency and loss of function. The causes of abnormal gait patterns vary according to the underlying pathology and may be skeletal or neuromuscular in nature. Neuromuscular pathology can involve the central nervous system or peripheral nerves. Some conditions can be progressive. An accurate diagnosis is necessary for the appropriate treatment and outcome. The pathology and its ramifications should be understood as a basis for treatment.

Pathomechanics is a branch of physical science that deals with the abnormal effects of static and dynamic forces on the human body affected by neurologic, muscular, and skeletal disorders. Pathologic gait is characterized by gait deviations, whereas pathomechanical gait addresses the underlying causes of the deviations. This distinction is crucial to the proper assessment of gait. It is important to determine the primary cause of a deviation rather than merely give it a name.

Simple guidelines should be followed for consistency among observers:

1. Observe gait with and without an existing orthosis (if applicable). An existing prosthesis can be compared with its replacement. Gait may be adversely affected by an inappropriate orthosis or prosthesis. Assistive devices or parallel bars should be used as required.
2. Look at the whole body first and get a general idea of the overall pattern. View from all planes (triplanar), and allow the patient to adjust to the fact that he or she is being observed. Have the patient walk initially without being filmed.
3. Single out areas of the body or segments of the gait to focus attention on the components of gait at each phase.
4. Begin to formulate an opinion as to the primary deficiency as opposed to compensations based on the knowledge of normal gait.
5. Perform gross functional muscle testing with the patient standing and supported in various postures. If the patient hyperextends the knee, can he or she support the weight on a flexed knee, or does he or she need the hyperextension for stability?

6. Acquire an overview of muscle tone, timing, and velocity. Muscle tone and other affectations of central nervous system pathology, such as ataxia and apraxia, should be recognized.
7. Allow for sufficient rest. Fatigue, anxiety, and fear affect the evaluation.

Physical examination

The purpose of the examination is to establish an inventory of physical deficiencies and the primary cause for each. The pattern of deficiencies creates an individual profile of the internal forces deranged by pathology, compensations, disuse, and premorbid condition. Movement is the primary concern, specifically as it relates to ambulation and the displacements noted in the mechanical evaluation.

Although it is necessary to perform a total body evaluation, it is not necessary to record normal function. In the examination, ROM and manual muscle testing (MMT) may be done separately, but cannot be isolated from each other. It is more meaningful to perform the ROM assessment and MMT for each joint at the same time. It is not necessary to grade each muscle. Muscle strength in the fair range (3) and below is more significant because gravity and GRF become more of an issue. Grades of normal and good (5 and 4) are significant only when there is an imbalance between two opposing muscle groups for a given joint and motion. While recording the deficiencies, attention should be given to the movement patterns as they relate to function [9].

Functional movement relates to the ability to complete the required pattern with sufficient force in a specific time frame for any given activity. Analyzing movement at a joint as a whole rather than in terms of ROM and strength has important treatment implications. Movement at the hips, knees, and ankles involves muscles that span two joints. These muscles must have sufficient length to allow the joint in question to complete the ROM required for the activity. Muscle length also is described as flexibility, indicating the ability of the muscle to be lengthened to the end of the ROM across the joint. Muscle length is of primary concern in human locomotion.

A differentiation should be made between passive ROM at a particular joint and muscle length. ROM at a particular joint is affected by bony joint surfaces, the joint capsule, muscles, and soft tissue or a combination thereof. Special consideration must be given to two joint muscles. According to Kendall et al, "For muscles that pass over one joint only, the ROM and range of muscle length will measure the same. For muscles that pass over two or more joints, the normal range of muscle length will be less than the total ROM of the joints over which the muscle passes" [10]. In functional movement, the limitation of joint ROM for two joint muscles depends on the joint that is stabilized. Stabilization of the proximal joint in the extended position becomes significant in treatment as it relates to gait.

Ultimately, the functional ROM allows for a movement pattern. Strength is a generic term that is used predominantly in rehabilitation. Strength refers to the ability of a muscle to develop force without reference to time. Muscles must develop peak force in milliseconds to be considered functional for a given activity; a more appropriate term is power because time is a specific requirement for function. Another important term is work. Work is defined as the application of force multiplied by the distance traveled. These terms are more functionally oriented as opposed to pure strength values. MMT is a useful tool, but it must be put in the proper perspective. It provides a baseline of information that serves as a guide for function; muscle test grades at isolated joints are obtained by having the clinician stabilize the joints proximal to the muscle being tested. The break test method allows the patient sufficient time to develop maximum force before resistance is applied by the clinician. In function, the patient must stabilize the proximal joint internally, and the force that a muscle group produces depends on time and distance traveled.

Gross testing of movement patterns can give insight into the more complex components of gait. Individual muscles and ROM at each joint need to be assessed; however, the combination of movement patterns required in gait places increased demands on strength and ROM. The ultimate goal is to allow for the movement pattern; in the treatment sequence, ROM is the primary consideration. Flexibility and muscle length must be considered as an important factor affecting ROM. Muscle balance is the next priority. Strength follows both in importance. Ultimately, the functional ROM allows for the completion of a movement pattern. Functional ROM incorporates ROM (muscle length), functional strength, and motor learning. A basic understanding of the neurophysiology of muscle function aids in the selection of treatment techniques.

The OrthoTherapy assessment protocol includes the following: ROM and MMT for the lower extremities, muscle length and flexibility testing, trunk and pelvic function, supplemental foot evaluation, sensory evaluation, an overview of the neck and upper extremities, and other pertinent and related information noted by the clinician. In the case of upper motor neuron involvement, a separate evaluation is performed.

Lower extremity range of motion and manual muscle testing

ROM and MMT are performed for the lower extremities. Normal and good (5 and 4) muscle grades and normal ROM are not charted. Joints with muscle grades of fair or less and incomplete ROM are reviewed more carefully. The limitations are charted along with the root cause. Notations are made for each movement at a joint, indicating muscle imbalance; asymmetry left/right; surgical fusions, coalitions, or contractures; and end feel of the range.

Passive ROM should be conducted with the subject completely relaxed with the joints stabilized and the lever arm securely held. As the joint approaches the end range, the trained practitioner can "feel" the manner in which the motion ends and the resistance, determining the primary cause of the limitation. These end feels are described in the following way [11]:

Bony: The motion ends abruptly. The resistance is hard and no further motion is possible. (B)

Capsular: The motion ends firmly. The resistance is firm but not hard. There is a very slight give to the movement. (C)

Muscular: The resistance is firm but springy. There is give to the movement. (M)

Soft tissue: The motion ends smoothly. The resistance is soft and mushy. (ST)

Pain: ROM is limited by pain (P)

The testing procedure itself is also an indication of the patient's physical status because the patient is required to change position frequently and expend energy in the process. How a patient moves should be noted and recorded. Muscle tone also should be assessed. In the case of upper motor neuron involvement, MMT is of limited value. Synergistic patterns of movement make muscle test grades invalid. Spasticity also affects ROM.

Muscle length and flexibility testing

Muscle length testing is performed on all of the two joint muscles of the lower extremity. The flexibility of these special muscles is one of the most important elements involved in functional movement patterns. The tests are listed subsequently. The clinician should review the information frequently until it becomes familiar. These tests are described in detail in the book by Reese and Brandy [11].

Iliopsoas muscle length is tested supine in the Thomas test position. Decreased muscle length of the iliopsoas is measured by the degree of hip flexion measured. A prone test measures the degree of hip extension (flexion).

Rectus femoris muscle length is tested supine in the Thomas test position or prone. Decreased muscle length of the rectus femoris is measured by the degree of knee flexion (extension).

Hamstring muscle length is tested supine in a straight-leg raise test, in which hip flexion is measured to determine length, or a knee extension test, in which maximum knee extension is measured.

Iliotibial band and tensor fascia latae muscle length is tested side lying with the Ober test or modified Ober test. This test is graded positive or negative. The hip remains abducted in a positive test and falls below horizontal in a negative test. A prone technique also can be performed.

Gastrocnemius muscle length is tested supine with the hip and knee in extension. Dorsiflexion of the foot is measured. It is crucial that the subtalar joint be maintained in a neutral position to test for true dorsiflexion. This is addressed in more detail in the supplemental foot evaluation.

Soleus muscle length is tested supine with the hip and knee in 45° of flexion. In the prone test, the hip is neutral, and the knee is flexed to 90°. Knee flexion relaxes the gastrocnemius muscle. Dorsiflexion is measured to determine soleus length. It is crucial to maintain a subtalar neutral position.

Trunk and pelvic function

As indicated in the section on kinesiology for clinicians, pelvic function plays a crucial role in the establishment of efficient gait. Along with ROM and muscle length, pelvic function becomes an important element in the treatment process. The rotary movements of the trunk and pelvis work together to create a smooth, fluid gait. The pelvis acts like a universal joint, whereas the trunk is the torque absorber. ROM is difficult to assess in these areas; the clinician must determine the degree of pelvic mobility and trunk flexibility.

Flexibility of the low back, pelvis, and upper trunk segments can be evaluated in the long sitting position (knees extended) or hook sitting position (knees flexed) depending on the degree of limitation. Tight extensor muscles, including the hamstrings, limit flexibility in flexing or reaching forward. Trunk extension can be assessed prone lying. The forward bend test (hands to floor) in the standing position provides similar information along with a sacroiliac evaluation. Pelvic mobility is tested in the following manner:

Supine: Pelvic tilt and elevation (sacral base tilt)
Side lying: Protraction and counterrotation (with trunk)
Prone: Low back and sacrum

Supplemental foot evaluation

In the section on kinesiology of normal locomotion, the foot/ankle complex is described as the foundation on which bipedal ambulation is made possible. In light of this statement, it is worth taking a closer look at this important component. The importance of the foot/ankle complex applies to the unilateral amputee and the individual with neuromuscular pathology. The amputee may have deficiencies in the remaining foot or ankle. The deficiency may be exacerbated by neuropathy or the increased stress on the normal side of the body. In either case, it is essential to evaluate the foot and ankle as a separate entity.

Inspection of the skin reveals bony anomalies, callus formation, any skin problems, and the degree of sensation. These are noted and recorded. An open chain evaluation of the foot determines the relationship of the talocrural joint, the midtarsal joint, and the forefoot and the existing ROM. Deformities are noted in addition to the degree of mobility and suppleness. The deformities vary from complete coalition or fusion (fixed deformities) to functional deformities that can be reduced to normal or near-normal conditions.

True dorsiflexion also must be established. Often "dorsiflexion" is obtained without regard to the relationship of the forefoot to the subtalar and midtarsal joints. In a pathomechanical foot that is not stable by virtue of ligamentous laxity or muscle weakness (absence), the forefoot is "dorsiflexed" with resultant calcaneal valgus and a collapse of the midtarsal joint. This is not true dorsiflexion. The proper method of testing is to perform the following sequence: plantar flex and invert the foot maximally; stabilize the calcaneus in a neutral position to avoid valgus and lock it in place; elevate the fifth ray of the forefoot, while maintaining a subtalar neutral position. In many instances, what appears to be dorsiflexion can be a plantar flexion contracture. Any orthotic system that does not take this into account would not be able to maintain the triplanar control necessary for balance and support; efficient gait is impossible.

A closed chain evaluation of the foot should be performed with the patient standing to determine the height of the heel lift necessary to accommodate for any existing contracture owing to an Achilles tendon shortening. With the patient standing in the anatomic position, the line of gravity (neutral plumb line) should pass from the knee center through the navicular, while maintaining a subtalar neutral position. This is the mandatory starting point for any orthotic system. If the contracture is functional in nature, a remodeling effect can be obtained through treatment and the proper application of an orthotic support system that maintains the neutrality of the subtalar and midtarsal joints.

Sensory evaluation

The sensory evaluation is an important element when dealing with neuropathy in an amputee or a patient with neuromuscular pathology. Superficial sensation is tested for light touch, pinprick, pressure, and temperature discrimination. Deep sensory or proprioception is tested for position (static), movement (kinesthesia), and vibration. Sensation awareness or lack thereof is an important element of treatment (education) and follow-up.

Neck and upper extremity evaluation

Because humans walk with their entire bodies, it is important not to overlook the influence of the neck and upper extremities on posture and gait. Deficiencies in any of these areas require further investigation and treatment.

Upper motor neuron evaluation for central nervous system involvement

If a patient shows upper motor neuron involvement secondary to head injury, cerebrovascular accident, or other central nervous system pathology, a supplemental evaluation is required to provide more reliable information. In cases of spasticity, MMT becomes invalid because synergistic movement patterns may be evident. Functional muscle testing is more appropriate in these cases. ROM remains a crucial factor especially with regard to velocity. Included in this evaluation are tests related to the following:

Cognition: The ability to follow directions; the ability to understand the task

Perception: Impulsive; distracted; frustrated; emotionally labile

Communication: Speech; language skills; auditory

Muscle tone: Reflexes; reciprocal motion (active and passive)

Coordination: Ataxia; apraxia; involuntary movements; initiation and force of movement

Balance and posture: Static; dynamic

Treatment plan

The purpose of the treatment plan is to establish the short-term and long-term goals necessary to achieve the intended outcome for an individual patient. It is the outline for treatment that includes the coordination of physical therapy and the provision of a prosthesis or an orthosis, combined with medical supervision. The roles of the prosthetist/orthotist and physical therapist overlap. The physician should continue to monitor the overall health and general well-being of the patient along with the use of appropriate medications. The patient must be medically stable to begin a rehabilitation program. Acute medical problems should be addressed before treatment.

The interrelationships between the mechanical and physical deficiencies established in the assessment are analyzed according to the layers of abnormal movements described by DynamicBracingSolutions. As indicated in the assessment, they relate to deformities that are structural in nature; deficiencies in neuromuscular function caused by muscle weakness, paralysis, or absence in the case of amputation; and compensations for balance of the head, arms, and trunk. In this way, the type and cause of the abnormal movement patterns can be determined. The focus of treatment is determined by the results of this analysis. The timing and coordination of treatment involving the prosthesis/orthosis also must be established.

The common goal for the physical therapist and the prosthetist/orthotist is functional ambulation that is efficient and as close to the normal parameters of normal gait as possible. To achieve this goal in the most time-efficient manner, several questions must be answered before treatment begins: What are the mechanical requirements of the patient? What can be done in physical therapy to improve the physical deficiencies of the patient? How will these changes affect the mechanical requirements? What type of mechanical system is most appropriate? When should the mechanical system be introduced into treatment? What physical requirements are imposed on the patient by the mechanical system? What must be done in physical therapy to prepare the patient for the specific technology being applied? If the patient already has been fitted with a prosthesis or an orthosis, does it meet all of the physical and mechanical requirements of the patient? How does gait training relate to the patient's physical and mechanical needs and the technology being applied? The treatment plan must answer these questions before treatment begins. The type of treatment, timing, and coordinated effort of the physical therapist and prosthetist/orthotist determine the results [12].

Short-term goals must be set in a methodical manner to accomplish interim and long-term goals. An example of a goal planning sequence would be to improve ROM or reduce a contracture at a particular joint or joints, improve or decrease a muscle imbalance, improve the functional movement pattern required as a component of efficient gait, and improve functional strength through repetition and practice of the activity.

Preprosthetic treatment is based on a series of short-term goals that prepares the patient for prosthetic fitting. Although preprosthetic treatment for the new amputee has long been established, it may or may not be performed in its entirety in the present health care delivery system. Considering the above-listed questions, all patients require preprosthetic assessment and treatment; this applies to long-term prosthetic wearers and new amputees. The same criteria apply in both cases; similarly, patients with neuromuscular pathologies require the same type of treatment. In contrast to prosthetics, this approach has never been shown consistently in orthotics.

How much of the outcome depends on physical therapy? How much of the outcome depends on the mechanical system? These questions cannot be answered in terms of percentages. They are simultaneously and equally important; the outcome depends on both. In the author's practice, the physical therapist and the prosthetist/orthotist are one and the same; it is easier for the author to look at both sides of the same treatment. Later tn the treatment section, the author provides some insight into the thought process necessary for the physical therapist and the prosthetist/orthotist to work together rather than separately. Everyone involved, including the patient, should be in complete agreement with the treatment plan.

Discussion of the plan and the commitment

When the treatment plan has been established, the intended outcome and the protocol of treatment are explained to the patient. Patients cannot be treated passively. They must become part of the treatment process. This requires their complete understanding, cooperation, and active participation. Expectations on the part of the patient and the clinician should be discussed openly and honestly. Any questions regarding treatment should be answered at this point rather than after the fact.

In the present health care system, treatment time and sessions are limited. Most of the treatment is conducted on an outpatient basis; it is important to make the most efficient use of time. Treatment sessions must be productive and educational to ensure carryover and good practice habits. Improvement and the ultimate outcome depend on the time and effort that the patient devotes to the program on his or her own. Even the most dedicated and experienced clinician cannot help patients more than they want to help themselves. The clinician merely provides the tools necessary for patients to help themselves. It is the patient's commitment to treatment that ultimately determines the outcome.

As part of the OrthoTherapy treatment protocol, the patient and the clinician sign a commitment agreement. This agreement outlines the responsibilities of the patient and the clinician. The clinician agrees to provide the necessary treatment to achieve the stated goals. This agreement includes the intended outcome; an appropriate prosthetic/orthotic system that guarantees the proper structural alignment, fit, and comfort (related to wearing tolerance); physical therapy treatment and training to coincide with the prosthesis/orthosis; and follow-up. The patient agrees to follow the protocol of treatment; devote the time and effort required to achieve the stated goals; consistently carry out a home program developed to coincide with scheduled treatment sessions; discuss any modifications to treatment with the clinician in advance; and seek the opinions of friends, family members, or other professionals before signing the agreement.

The clinician and the patient are dependent on each other for the successful outcome of treatment. It is truly a team effort. Any doubt or hesitation on the part of the patient should be reason *not* to proceed. On completion of the commitment agreement, treatment can begin with a positive attitude. A positive attitude generates positive results.

Treatment

OrthoTherapy methodology and guidelines

So far, this article has examined the outcome and the assessment based on an understanding of the kinesiology of normal (efficient) posture and ambulation and pathomechanical (inefficient) gait considerations. The physical and mechanical profiles established for each patient outline the internal deficiencies that need to be addressed in physical therapy and the requirements of the external mechanical system. The forces acting on the body during ambulation include GRF, inertia (acceleration), and gravity (COG). Corrective forces include body position, muscular control, and external mechanical system. With a better understanding of the elements involved and their relationship to one another, clinicians can reconstruct them in the treatment process to build the framework necessary to achieve the intended outcome. As mentioned in the discussion on outcomes, efficiency in gait can be achieved only through the motor learning process.

Skilled voluntary movements and the implications for gait training and treatment

The kinesiology of posture, ambulation, and movement therapy are essential ingredients in the successful treatment plan. Successful treatment implies that movement is not only purposeful and efficient, but also automatic and instinctive. It is important that clinicians understand the underlying principles of teaching and learning motor skills.

Voluntary movement implies that a conscious decision is made to initiate and perform activities. Many movement patterns make up the activity. Inhibition of muscle groups is as significant as excitation. Nonessential movements must be inhibited as the prime movers or agonistic muscle groups guide the activity. (This applies to the mechanical system and internal muscle control.) In many cases, there is a cocontraction about a joint to create stability or controlled movement in one direction. Initiation of the action is voluntary and under cortical control. In skilled activity, performance of the act is automatic and subcortically controlled; the individual is unaware of the components of movement patterns that compose the activity. New activities can be learned only with persistent effort and repeated trials. Skill implies that the activity becomes automatic. Walking efficiently is a highly skilled activity and occurs only after numerous complex motor patterns have been mastered in a developmental sequence.

Normal ambulation involves the coordinated effort of the entire body. This is a learned activity that requires confidence. It appears to be one continuous motion, but in actuality, it is a complex series of movement patterns. For amputees and individuals with pathomechanical deficiencies, this series of patterns must be relearned.

With the outcome in mind, one must start at the beginning. What is required to achieve an efficient gait pattern? The objective is to begin ambulation as soon as possible with the stipulation that all the prerequisites are met methodically and in the proper sequence. The primary requirement is standing (static) balance. Balance is reflected in posture. The effects of gravity and GRF combined with physical deficiencies affect posture and balance. Primary physical deficiencies include amputation, limitations in ROM and muscle length, muscle imbalance with associated weakness or paralysis, and spasticity.

Compensations during ambulation are normal responses to the lack of balance and the fear of falling. These compensations are referred to as gait deviations. Deviations are not deformities, but voluntary movement patterns that become automatic over time in response to security issues. Compensations are secondary to primary physical and mechanical deficiencies. The objective is to treat problems rather than symptoms. Left untreated, the primary problems lead to deformity.

Based on this information, gait training takes on a different meaning. A patient cannot simply be told what to do to correct a deviation or improve the gait pattern. Appropriate movement patterns must be learned. In this context, gait training has several phases, including gait preparation, gait awareness, and gait practice. Gait preparation involves physical therapy treatment to improve physical deficiencies. Gait awareness combines these internal corrective forces with the external mechanical device. Gait practice is the positive reinforcement of the appropriate movement patterns required for efficient ambulation. Negative reinforcement has the opposite effect. "Practice makes perfect" only if it is done properly.

Treatment must follow a logical sequence that adheres to a consistent philosophy. The primary concern in OrthoTherapy is movement and the application to prosthetic/orthotic technology. In the assessment section, common terms used in the physical examination were modified in keeping with this philosophy; likewise, the term exercise becomes movement therapy. Strengthening and stretching are replaced with power training and flexibility. This is more than just semantics. It is part of the methodology that establishes a specific way of thinking about treatment.

The methodology and the sequence (timing) are crucial components of treatment. The effectiveness of treatment is determined by the application of the corrective forces relative to the external forces acting on the body during ambulation. In biomechanical treatment, the internal forces of the patient and the mechanical forces of the prosthesis/orthosis must be combined. The key to treatment is the pelvis and its relationship to the trunk proximally and the lower extremities distally. Body position and muscular control are the corrective forces that represent the bio aspect of treatment. These are examined first.

Bio (physical) treatment: gait preparation

The short-term goals are to treat the primary physical deficiencies that relate to static balance. ROM and muscle flexibility are the primary concerns. The most common physical problem related to pelvic function is decreased muscle length followed by muscle imbalance. Decreased iliopsoas flexibility causes an increased lumbar lordosis and a functional hip flexion contracture. If hip extension is tested without regard to pelvic stabilization, it may appear to be normal; as a result, hip extension is obtained with an anteriorly tilted pelvis or increased lumbar lordosis. The compensatory trunk position causes a shortening of the low back muscles, resulting in muscle imbalance with weak stretched abdominals and strong tight extensors. This swayback posture also favors decreased flexibility in the hamstrings and weak gluteal muscles. This is a common problem in the general population and may be a premorbid condition in many cases, exacerbated by amputation or other pathology.

To neutralize the pelvis in this situation, the hip must flex. Pelvic stabilization in the neutral position is the ultimate goal. Muscle length must be increased to improve ROM. As ROM increases, muscle imbalance can be addressed. If the opposing muscle group is nonfunctional, ROM must be increased to a functional degree, and the lack of muscle control must be replaced by an external force system in the form of a prosthesis or an orthosis. These are the initial goals of treatment.

Preambulation exercises and gait training are basic rehabilitation treatment procedures. Traditionally, they have been separated in the treatment plan, with a mat program designed to prepare the patient for ambulation followed by gait training. Gait preparation combines these procedures. The exercises are performed on a mat table and follow a developmental sequence beginning with activities with a large BOS and a low COG, progressing to activities with a smaller BOS and a higher COG. The elimination of gravity avoids the negative reinforcement caused by compensations. As each separate movement becomes imprinted, the movements are connected to form the appropriate movement patterns. Only then can they be positively reinforced while standing and ambulating [13].

The mat program follows the four stages of motor control:

1. Mobility: The therapist may assist the initiation of movement patterns. The patient learns the movement, posture, and position.
2. Stability: This involves the ability to maintain a posture against gravity or to stabilize a proximal joint for the appropriate movement pattern of distal joints.
3. Controlled mobility: This is the ability to maintain postural control during weight shifting and movement.
4. Skill: This implies discrete motor control superimposed on proximal stability.

Except in severe neuromuscular cases, it is not necessary to follow the complete sequence. In OrthoTherapy, the mat program is used primarily to improve body awareness in a nongravity situation to emphasize basic movement patterns necessary for ambulation; pelvic rotation can be simulated in rolling activities. This training forms the basis for learning more complex movement patterns, such as counterrotation of the trunk and pelvis. In this way, the patient can experience the components of more complex patterns of motion in isolation and then build on them. It is difficult to feel a movement until it is experienced consciously. Conscious control of movement must be limited to one component at a time until it becomes automatic. Awareness and precise execution of the movement is the goal, following the four stages of motor control.

Mat work can be combined with therapeutic exercise. Proprioceptive neuromuscular facilitation is a good method to increase ROM, facilitate movement patterns, improve muscle balance, and enhance stability. Proprioceptive neuromuscular facilitation techniques are based on triplanar diagonal movement patterns and offer more functional value than progressive resistive exercises [14].

Interim goals may be established to concentrate on physical therapy before or in combination with ambulation. This decision is based on the number and degree of physical deficiencies present; a transtibial amputee may have decreased length in the iliopsoas and rectus femoris muscles. These deficiencies reduce ROM, causing hip and knee flexion contractures resulting in muscle imbalance with stronger flexion and weaker extension at the hip and knee. In this case, short-term goals to improve muscle length, ROM, and muscle balance would precede prosthetic fitting because these deficiencies would preclude the movement patterns necessary for balance. Caution should be exercised not to exceed the patient's ability to assume and control the posture. Work should be done at the lowest level at which the movement can be completed.

When the elements for balance have been established, gait preparation and gait practice can be done together. Ambulation may continue in a progressive manner, while mat activities can revert to more basic movements for emphasis. Each patient is different not only in terms of deficiencies, but also in natural abilities. Some patients are referred to as "naturals" because they have a more developed sense of body awareness, agility, or coordination. Others require more practice. Treatments necessarily vary. Even good ambulators require mat work and movement therapy to improve pelvic mobility and stabilization to achieve greater efficiency [15].

Pilates connection

Because mobility is based on a stable base, lumbar stabilization has always been a consideration in a good therapeutic exercise program. In hindsight, it was simply part of the treatment and was not given the special attention it deserved. In the Pilates method of exercise, it is the centerpiece of physical movement. On a personal level, Pilates is the final piece of the puzzle that changed the way the author views the completed picture. It has put all of the author's past experience in perspective and has provided a better understanding of how all of the elements of treatment are related to form the whole. The author's interest in Pilates led to a mat certification program for physical therapists and has become a guiding factor in Ortho-Therapy treatment.

Pilates is a mind-body exercise philosophy that emphasizes core strengthening in movement training. In contrast to the large external muscles of the trunk represented by the rectus abdominis (flexion) and longissimus dorsi (extension), the smaller internal muscles are emphasized. These include, but are not limited to, transversus abdominis, multifidus, interspinales, and pyramidalis. The primary role of these muscles is stabilization and does not include the production of motion. They are responsible for controlling posture. Without this function, the large external muscles are overworked and become tighter and stronger. This causes the inner stabilizing muscle to become stretched and weak. This provides a better understanding of the relationship between the limitations in ROM and muscle imbalance on the most basic level. Without this internal stabilization, posture and balance are adversely affected. Exercising the large outer muscle groups to achieve stability only increases the problem.

Pilates methodology and terminology have changed since Joseph Pilates first developed his program. It has become more scientific and related to the principles of therapeutic exercise and rehabilitation. Originally, the core was referred to as the powerhouse of the body with all activity emanating from the center. A vigorous flat back posture was emphasized for all body types.

Modern Pilates emphasizes exercising in a neutral spine position and has been described earlier as the vertical line connecting the symphysis pubis and the anterior superior iliac spine. All movement is performed in this position, and the goal is to gain strength and length while moving away from the center. Lengthening while you strengthen refers to the ability to produce movement patterns away from the center, while maintaining stability in the neutral spine position. The objective of the movement is to complete the range with precision while maintaining a neutral spine. Control and ROM are crucial. By stabilizing the core, true ROM may be limited as compensations in the spine and extremities are eliminated; it is necessary to work within the confines of a neutral spine to increase ROM [16].

Overstretching in an attempt to increase ROM results in the loss of the neutral spine position, which adversely affects posture and balance. Excessive resistance or strength training also is counterproductive because it encourages limited ROM and further muscle imbalance. In such cases, already strong muscle groups get stronger and tighter, while weaker muscle groups get weaker and more stretched. These are common errors of exercise made with good intentions. The mind-body connection forces the individual to concentrate on the proper components of movement. Performed correctly over time, they become automatic.

Pilates also emphasizes scapular stabilization. Postural control requires the shoulders to be in the ideal plumb line; this maintains the trunk in the proper alignment. The phrase wrapping the shoulder blades implies a sense of gently sliding the scapulae down and back without forcing them. This is the starting position for all upper extremity movement. The method used to achieve the neutral spine position is called scooping the abdominals. This visualization is an important part of Pilates. It is used to enhance movement and can be helpful in gait training. When a patient stands they immediately scoop the abdomen, wrap the shoulder blades, and look straight ahead with the head up and back to assume the proper posture. The objective is to stand tall [17].

Breathing is a topic that is discussed in every reference to exercise as the foundation for movement; it is rarely incorporated into treatment. Most people do not know how to breathe properly. This too must be learned. Siphon breathing involves the use of the chest muscles, whereas piston breathing primarily involves the diaphragm. Both of these types of breathing are inefficient because they limit vital capacity. Lateral breathing or bellows breathing makes full use of the lung capacity, as the rib cage moves downward and outward on inspiration. Vital capacity is an important part of endurance training and should not be overlooked [18].

Although Pilates is a method of exercise in its own right, it can be included in biomechanical treatment combined with other therapeutic exercise techniques. Movement therapy should include techniques to establish co-contraction for active joint stabilization; the use of slow, controlled, closed kinetic chain exercises; focus on joint position; emphasis on positioning tasks that require precision and control; use of low force levels for training; and activities that challenge balance as ROM and muscle balance improve. Movement therapy should avoid high strength training and overexercising of the large torque-producing muscles. This avoidance coincides with the philosophy of treatment that emphasizes ROM and muscle length first, followed by muscle balance with core stabilization as the basis for treatment. This philosophy applies to athletes and patients beginning a rehabilitation program. Efficiency in normal subjects can be improved with this method.

Home program: continuity of treatment

It is not possible to accomplish treatment goals without the development of a home program of movement therapy designed to reinforce and facilitate sessions with the clinician. These sessions might include a hands-on mat program emphasizing core stability and movement patterns that lengthen and strengthen. Pilates exercises are a good way to acquaint patients with their center and teach proper breathing essential for appropriate exercise. This can be combined with other therapeutic exercise techniques, such as proprioceptive neuromuscular facilitation. Treatment with an exercise ball (Swiss ball) also can be effective. An innovative physical therapist can apply various techniques to accomplish the same purpose. These techniques form the basis for the home program that allows the patient to continue to improve on his or her own.

Ultimately, the patient must be responsible for his or her own treatment, which is a condition of the commitment agreement. Professional guidance and education are primary objectives of treatment. As patients learn the appropriate movement patterns and techniques to improve physical deficiencies, they must be reinforced on a daily basis. The results depend on the time and effort applied to the task. There must be carryover from one session to the next. To make the most efficient use of treatment time, the clinician reviews and reinforces the home program so that progress is ongoing.

Mechanical system

The ability to balance has physical and mechanical components. The posture necessary for balance is obtained by correcting or improving the existing physical deficiencies (internal force) combined with an appropriate prosthetic/orthotic system (external force). Together they allow for appropriate body position.

Although the goal of gait preparation is to correct or improve physical deficiencies, it is important to realize what can and cannot be achieved with physical therapy alone. Any physical improvement would reduce the demands placed on the mechanical system; residual weakness or absence of muscle function can be replaced only with an appropriate prosthetic/orthotic system. This third corrective force must replace missing function that cannot be restored internally.

The mechanical system provides the triplanar alignment and support in combination with the internal forces necessary for balance. Starting from the ground up, the anterior foot lever (prosthetic or orthotic) must be sufficient in terms of the GRF to support the proximal joints (anatomic or mechanical) in the proper alignment in the sagittal plane without excessive muscle effort. Alignment in the frontal plane also should provide for mediolateral (ML) stability, allowing body position to remain midline without the need for compensations. Rotary forces must be controlled in the transverse plane to maintain alignment, stability, and momentum.

Although this alignment applies to prosthetics and orthotics equally, it is inherently more difficult in orthotics. The prosthetist can alter the alignment of the external prosthetic components at any time during the fitting procedure. The orthotist must realign the internal skeletal components to achieve the intended result during the casting and modification procedures. The foot must be controlled distally, while rotation is controlled proximally. Appropriate design and materials application complete the mechanical elements needed to provide support, maintain alignment, and control internal forces through GRF. Triplanar control is required to align the skeletal and external components, which is a prerequisite for balance. Correction in one or even two planes of motion is insufficient.

Orthotic treatment must focus on the specific neuromuscular pathology in addition to the mechanics of the system. Deficiencies and loss of function related to the primary pathology need to be identified and isolated from muscle weakness resulting from disuse or compensations. Residual weakness or paralysis requires the corrective force of the mechanical system, whereas weakness caused by disuse or compensations can be treated with physical therapy. The individual pattern of this combined weakness and loss of function makes orthotic treatment challenging. Generally, prosthetic treatment is more mechanical in nature and deals primarily with muscle weakness from disuse or compensations. In such cases, physical therapy is indicated; however, patients with secondary diagnoses, such as neuropathy, present similar neuromuscular concerns. In all cases, premorbid physical deficiency also is a factor. This deficiency should be identified and treated accordingly. Individual patterns of combined muscle weakness vary, as should effective treatment.

The laws of mechanics that have been applied to prosthetic technology need to be applied equally to orthotics. As prosthetic technology has improved, orthotic technology has been stagnant. Most orthoses treat symptoms rather primary deficiencies. Dropfoot braces solve a swing phase problem without addressing stance phase support or triplanar alignment for stability. Many of the new swing phase devices are prefabricated and serve only one purpose. Two notable exceptions are the development of dynamic response rotary control orthoses and stance control knee joints. Stance control knees are only one component of a mechanical system. Although extremely valuable, this component is affected by design and materials. Stance control (support) is important in every orthosis, including ankle-foot orthoses. In many cases, design and materials can offer support to weak muscles through GRF without orthotic knee joints. Orthoses must be re-examined as mechanical systems designed for function rather than symptomatic relief. "An orthosis must be viewed as combining with body parts to form a mechanical system that obeys mechanical laws and achieves mechanical effects" [3]. The role of the clinician is to make certain that the mechanical effect is the intended effect.

It is important to consider the design and materials in the mechanical system and how these elements relate to support, alignment, and balance. An orthotic example might be a polypropylene ankle-foot orthosis with a posterior cuff for a patient with proximal weakness. The support in this case is in the wrong place relative to GRF. The material is too flexible and would deform under load. There is no rotary control. In this example, the mechanical system is working against the already weak internal forces. A more appropriate mechanical design would provide pretibial support combined with the proper foot lever to prevent excessive hip and knee flexion during stance phase. To accomplish this, a more rigid material is required.

A prosthetic example might be a transtibial amputee with a large, soft residual limb who has an ML instability problem in a standard patellar tendon bearing (PTB) socket. Alignment of the distal components depends on proximal stability. Supracondylar design is a consideration because it provides support, stability, and suspension. A well-contoured proximal brim provides the counterforce necessary to maintain proper alignment. For purposes of discussion, it is assumed that fit is appropriate; however, this assumption should not be made in treatment.

These examples illustrate the need to isolate and anticipate problems that exist in the mechanical system before ambulation begins. The corrective force applied by the mechanical system must work in harmony with body position and muscle control to create the intended effect. This begins the gait awareness phase of treatment.

Biomechanical treatment

Gait awareness

When static balance is achieved, the next goal is dynamic balance, which involves the shifting of the COG in all planes of motion, while maintaining a stationary foot placement. This movement is performed initially with the feet together followed by a diagonal stance with one foot in front of the other (then reversed); this allows the patient to explore the extreme points of balance with the mechanical system. After this movement, but before ambulation, the stance phase transitions of weight acceptance and stance limb progression on the mechanical system are broken down. First, the prosthesis/orthosis is placed in front of the other foot to simulate weight acceptance (heel contact to midstance). With the pelvis in the neutral position, the COG is shifted forward to midstance or single limb support. Stability and balance are tested in this position. Next, the prosthesis/orthosis is placed behind the other foot to simulate stance limb progression (from midstance to heel-off). With the pelvis in the neutral position, the COG is shifted forward from midstance to terminal stance to test the foot lever relative to knee stability; this is repeated on both sides for bilateral involvement.

Dynamic balance exercises apply to orthotic and prosthetic cases and serve to evaluate the mechanical system in terms of alignment and support. The foot levers are tested relative to the timing and duration of support in early and late stance. All mechanical systems are floor reaction devices [19]. This is an excellent time to familiarize the patient with the mechanical system. Stance control components (prosthetic and orthotic) rely on the forward movement of the COG over the foot lever to disengage stance control in preparation for swing phase. Stance control in a transtibial prosthesis or an ankle-foot orthosis requires the mechanical system to provide a lever system using GRF to replace or assist the eccentric contraction of the knee extensors during stance phase. Hip extension is the physical counterforce or corrective force that must be incorporated into the movement pattern. A transtibial amputee may have normal strength, but has a functional weakness owing to the loss of leverage. In both cases, the support needs to be anterior, and the material should be sufficiently rigid to prevent rotation in the transverse plane and maintain alignment stability in the frontal plane, while allowing for movement or flexibility in the sagittal plane. This allows for dynamic balance in stance phase and eliminates the need to hyperextend the knee for security reasons.

Similarly, the patient needs to be aware of the foot component (prosthetic or orthotic) and how the GRF affects support and stability. In the gait awareness phase of treatment, all of the corrective forces must be examined, as they relate to the function of the whole biomechanical system. It is essential that any deficiencies in the mechanical system be made before proceeding with gait practice. Based on knowledge of motor learning, the goal of the practice sessions is to provide positive reinforcement of the appropriate movement patterns repeatedly so that they become automatic. In this way, confidence is established, which sets the stage for continued improvement.

Gait practice

The goal of the gait practice phase of treatment is to integrate the internal forces of muscular control and body position with the external mechanical system. Because gait practice involves the whole system, physical and mechanical treatment often coincide. The most efficient use of time demands that specific deficiencies in gait be treated appropriately; in other words, is physical or mechanical treatment required or a combination of both? Who decides what needs to be done? The physical therapist and the prosthetist/orthotist must work together for a sufficient period to think like one clinician. As a prerequisite for success, everyone needs to be in agreement with the treatment plan. There cannot be separate opinions, and no one is more important than another. Everyone involved must understand the scientific basis for treatment. The role of the team is to make adjustments in treatment as determined by the deficiencies observed and to guide the patient in the motor learning process.

Feedback is an important part of gait practice. Mirrors are useful for balance activities and a frontal view of the gait pattern, but they have limited value. Videotaping of practice sessions is an excellent learning tool. Patients are unaware of how they walk. Seeing themselves on tape can be a revelation. Anterior, posterior, and lateral views show all aspects of the gait cycle. The use of slow motion and stop motion can be effective in the educational process. The immediate feedback reinforces the feeling of movement with the actual movement itself. In this way, the patient can see the deficiency and the correction required in addition to the improvement.

Video analysis of inefficient gait often reveals a monolithic pattern in which the trunk and pelvis seem fused. There is a lack of counterrotation between the trunk and pelvis. The shoulders remain parallel to the hips as measured by a line connecting each anterior superior iliac spine. Arm swing is limited. The pelvis is often tilted anteriorly in the sagittal plane, with an increased lumbar lordosis; this causes the trunk to lean forward, which causes compensatory upper trunk extension. In the frontal plane, the pelvis may not be horizontal owing to excessive weight shifting to one side, causing the trunk to lean laterally; this should not be confused with a leg-length discrepancy. In the transverse plane, the pelvis may rotate inappropriately or not at all. Forward motion is interrupted with movements that are up, down, sideways, and backward. This movement represents a net decrease in efficiency. The subject appears to be leading with the head and shoulders.

The causes of inefficient gait must be recognized and avoided in treatment. The best technology provided at the wrong time without appropriate preparation and awareness does not optimize the intended outcome. The effectiveness of gait practice lies in the details, rather than in the overt act of walking. Every patient has different needs based on their physical profile. Some have more natural ability than others, whereas some may have existing habits based on previous experience with an inappropriate mechanical system. If compensations have become normal, new movement patterns feel awkward to the patient even if they are more efficient. Old habits feel more comfortable. The level of proficiency required for the corrective movement patterns can be assessed on the mat, and physical treatment should coincide with gait practice. The goal is to increase efficiency for every patient regardless of the starting point. A good gait pattern does not imply one that is efficient. Gait practice in these cases can be more challenging because the details are harder to define and treat.

Putting the pieces together

Effective gait practice is based on a forward strategy. Balance is the foundation, and the focus is on pelvic function and how it relates to the trunk and lower extremities. As the trunk inclines forward to initiate a step, the pelvis must move forward in the neutral position to place the COG over the point of support as quickly as possible during the loading response. In visual terminology, the pelvis leads the way and must reach the finish line ahead of all other body parts. The symmetry and timing of the gait cycle maintain dynamic balance and the momentum necessary for a sustainable velocity. If the corrective forces are optimal, guidance is all that is needed. The methodology of a forward strategy follows the sequence described earlier: balance, pelvic function, symmetry, timing, velocity, and momentum. These gait characteristics can be compared with the video analysis to reinforce treatment.

As the patient stands from the seated position, a mental routine can assist in assuming the correct posture before ambulation begins. Through repetition, this posture becomes automatic. Using pelvic positioning with core stabilization (Pilates), the patient puts the feet together, scoops the abdomen and moves the hips forward over the feet, wraps the scapulae and moves the shoulders back, keeps the head up and eyes forward, shifts the weight to midline, takes a deep lateral breath, and relaxes. Over time, this procedure can be simplified with the visualization of standing tall. The verbal cue is to assume the stance.

The initiation of movement with the first step is crucial. As the trunk inclines forward, the pelvis must move forward. A common deviation is vaulting; this is caused by upward movement of the COG and is inefficient and energy-consuming. The first step must be practiced repeatedly. The patient decides which foot to move first, then inclines the trunk with the pelvis moving forward rather than up. The patient literally falls forward. The visualization is that of a swan dive where the hips lead the movement. In the gait cycle, the foot stops the fall. A stabilized core with the pelvis in the neutral position prevents trunk and hip flexion. Dynamic balance must be re-established with the hips leading the movement, while keeping the shoulders back.

The pelvis should be the focus of attention. Every movement of the lower extremities and trunk should be performed in the stabilized position. The pelvis (COG) must move forward to cause hip extension. Hip extension in itself is meaningless in the motor learning process. According to Beevor's axiom, "the brain knows nothing of individual muscle action but knows only of movement" [14]. In keeping with this axiom, guidance by the clinician should emphasize the movement of the pelvis.

Pelvic rotation and counterrotation between the trunk and pelvis is often reduced or absent. The matwork in gait preparation can be reinforced standing by having the patient assume the stance. First, the patient moves the right hip forward. The left shoulder is then moved forward. This movement is repeated on the left. The movements must be done separately until they feel natural. Only then can the movements be combined. This movement can be reinforced in gait with a relaxed arm swing, but the motion is initiated by the pelvis, not the arms.

The anterior superior iliac spine on each side can be likened to headlights of a car that must shine in the LOP. The driving force of the leg is established with a stabilized pelvis that is continually moving forward. With left heel contact, the right anterior superior iliac spine is driving forward and reverses with a right heel contact. This alternating movement of the pelvis is the force behind counterrotation because the trunk has a more passive role and must be relaxed. These pelvic movements give the appearance of stability.

Symmetry of step lengths also is lacking in inefficient gait patterns, resulting in reduced stride length. The tendency is to take a longer step with the involved side and a shorter step on the contralateral side; this increases swing time and reduces stance time on the orthosis or prosthesis. To increase stance phase on the mechanical device, the patient is instructed to think about the contralateral extremity, not the mechanical device. The patient should think one step ahead; the instant before the foot on the mechanical device contacts the floor, the patient should step out with the trailing leg moving the pelvis forward as quickly as possible. The command is to take a quicker and longer step, ignoring the mechanical device. Concentration on the prosthesis or orthosis is counterproductive in this case. Verbal cuing to take a shorter step with the mechanical device can be confusing and detracts from the forward strategy. Symmetry in the gait cycle is a prerequisite for increased velocity.

To quantify symmetry for outcomes, measurements must be taken. In practice sessions, the goal is to establish the symmetry through timing. To achieve equal step lengths, step times also must be equal; if the emphasis is on step times, symmetry also is improved. A metronome is a simple tool that serves this purpose well. The number of beats per minute is set to simulate a comfortable walking speed for the patient. Each heel contact must match the beat of the metronome. The goal is to develop a rhythm that establishes a uniform cadence. A treadmill also serves this purpose, but is not as simple to use and may not be available.

Momentum or acceleration is a force that must be considered in gait practice. The force is generated by the continuous forward movement of the pelvis (COG in the LOP). Any interruptions in this forward movement in the form of deviations or asymmetry detract from this force. Without this force, a sustainable velocity is impossible. The long-term goal of gait practice is to increase endurance with efficient movement that is fluid and relaxed.

Deficiencies in the gait pattern should be related to one or more of the corrective forces and treated accordingly. The internal forces of muscle control and body position may require reinforcement with additional mat work or therapeutic exercise in combination with gait practice. This requirement must be considered before changes are made to the mechanical system; if the mechanical system does not provide the proper support or alignment necessary for dynamic balance throughout the gait cycle, changes are in order.

The polypropylene ankle-foot orthosis with a posterior cuff lacks support for weak proximal musculature and causes increased flexion moments at the hip and knee at heel contact through GRF. This situation is inappropriate, and the mechanical system needs to be redesigned to provide anterior support in combination with improved design and materials. Muscles weakened by the primary pathology must be supported by the orthosis. This situation also can occur in well-designed systems. A prosthesis with an energy-storing carbon foot with a high activity (impact) level causes similar moments of force. The hip extensors must produce the counterforce necessary to maintain the hip and knee in the proper position throughout the gait cycle. A stabilized pelvis with sufficient core strength is a prerequisite. The foot may be too stiff, or the corrective force of muscular control needs to be increased. All mechanical systems are part of the biomechanical system and require active muscle control to function properly. Internal muscle counterforce is necessary for the intended function of the technology being used.

Gait practice depends on a mechanical system that is properly designed and well fitted to create the intended effect; however, it is important to recognize the effect of volume changes on fit and stability. As volume decreases in the anatomic or residual limb, total contact is lost, and unwanted movement of the limb occurs within the mechanical device. This movement destroys the intimacy needed to maintain the established alignment. The crucial balance of the corrective forces and counterforces is altered. Unchecked, this altered balance adversely affects gait practice.

The first recourse is to adjust the interface material. Total contact in prosthetics and orthotics is essential. Increasing the number of ply of the socks is a simple adjustment but is often overlooked. Fit determines function and comfort. In such cases, alignment changes do not solve the deficiencies caused by volume changes. If sock adjustment does not restore the original fit, further adjustments are required by the prosthetist/orthotist. Patients should be instructed to carry a change of socks at all times and make adjustments promptly when needed. True suction sockets in transfemoral prostheses are an exception because adjustments may be more involved.

Some general guidelines make gait practice more effective. It is important to give one command at a time. If this does not work, try another. Two or more commands cannot be assimilated. Keep it simple. Patients cannot think and walk at the same time. The body must learn the activity, but first the patient must be conscious of the proper movement patterns before they can become automatic; the patient must feel the movement as it is performed. The mechanical system should be explained to the patient. The patient must develop trust and confidence. Proper breathing and relaxation are important. The gait pattern cannot be forced or rigid.

Although safety is a primary concern, the use of assistive devices alters the gait pattern. Efficiency in gait cannot be obtained with a walker or crutches because they interfere with the forward strategy. Canes can be used to maintain the body in midline, but the primary objective is to increase efficiency and eliminate the need for assistive devices. Assistive devices impose forces on the biomechanical system that may be counterproductive to the intended outcome.

Treatment must be viewed by its physical and mechanical elements simultaneously. Only then can the appropriate action be taken. In general, the prosthetist/orthotist treats the patient from the ground up (distal to proximal), whereas the physical therapist treats the patient from proximal to distal. An established team can treat the whole biomechanical system.

Follow-up and future plan

The treatment plan is designed to improve the efficiency of ambulation. The best exercise is to walk appropriately and efficiently. Progress depends on the continuation of positively reinforced movement patterns that ensure efficiency in the gait pattern. When the patient is discharged from active treatment, follow-up visits should be scheduled to monitor the status of the whole biomechanical system and the need for changes in the physical or mechanical components. Patients must learn what they can do on their own and what requires the attention of the prosthetist/orthotist, the physical therapist, or the physician. Six-month follow-up visits are optimal followed by yearly visits. These visits are intended to insure that progress is ongoing. The goal of treatment is to improve the efficiency of ambulation. The ultimate goal of rehabilitation is to improve the quality of life.

It is recommended that each patient participate in a fitness program in combination with a healthy lifestyle that includes good nutrition and general health maintenance. There are many low-impact exercise programs for people of any age. Pilates and yoga are examples. In some cases, the two are combined to enhance physical and mental well-being [20]. It is important to focus on mobility and flexibility because these are the primary requirements for functional activity. Fitness should be fun. Movement is the main objective. It is not necessary to exercise or stretch. It could be detrimental if done improperly. Cardiovascular fitness is another concern. Cardiovascular fitness applies to everyone, including amputees and individuals with neuromuscular pathology. Preexisting cardiac problems must be monitored by a physician. Biomechanical treatment should prepare the patient for all activities of life in general. Efficient ambulation is the way to get there.

Summary

Biomechanical treatment is like a jigsaw puzzle with two complex counterparts having many pieces. The physical and mechanical components are equally important and cannot be separated from each other. The patient with a prosthesis or an orthosis represents a biomechnaical system; total treatment is essential. All of the pieces to the puzzle must be used to complete the picture.

Given the present structure of the educational system, there is a separation of disciplines necessary to provide one truly biomechanical treatment. Physical therapists are educated in the bio aspect of treatment, whereas prosthetists/orthotists are educated in the mechanical aspect. Biomechanical treatment requires the direct interaction and integration of the two disciplines. Physical therapists and prosthetists/orthotists need each other. One without the other can provide only half of the treatment necessary for optimal outcomes. The patient needs both.

Physical therapists need to become more familiar with mechanical treatment and learn how to integrate this into their physical treatment program. Prosthetists/orthotists must become more familiar with the importance of physical treatment and the internal corrective forces necessary for efficient ambulation. The traditional label of orthotics and prosthetics and related technology as products must be replaced with biomechanical treatment that includes orthotics and prosthetics services.

Professionals working with each other is a positive step, but they need to be working together as a team toward a common goal. They need to be in the same place at the same time and work together consistently to provide total treatment. This is more than a multidisciplinary approach. It is one treatment. In this way, each benefits the other as they teach and learn simultaneously. At present, this teaching and learning can be done only on an individual basis.

It is the author's hope that experienced prosthetists/orthotists and physical therapists reading this article will see the need to combine their efforts to provide truly biomechanical treatment. By working together, they can expand their present knowledge and skills. In this way, treatment and outcomes can improve and serve as the guiding force for a new generation of rehabilitation specialists. This process can be expedited through the educational system by offering advanced clinical degrees specializing in biomechanical treatment specifically designed for clinical practice rather than research, administrative, or academic positions. For this idea to become reality, educational institutions representing the physical and mechanical aspects of biomechanical treatment also must work together; this would expedite the learning curve so that it would not take so long to put the pieces of the puzzle together.

Acknowledgments

The author is indebted to Jean-Paul Nielsen and Marmaduke Loke for their experience and teaching in advanced orthotic design and technology.

As rehabilitation specialists and the creators of DynamicBracingSolutions, they have applied the scientific principles of mechanics and pathomechanics to orthotic support systems. These systems treat the primary deficiencies of pathology and related compensations, providing the appropriate mechanical component of treatment. In combination with the physical component, comprehensive biomechanical treatment is possible in orthotics and prosthetics. My education in DynamicBracingSolutions stimulated my interest as a physical therapist and was a major influence in the development of OrthoTherapy.

References

[1] Craik RL, Oatis CA. The neurophysiology of human locomotion. In: Gait analysis theory and application. St. Louis: Mosby; 1995. p. 47.
[2] Merriam-Webster's Collegiate Dictionary. Springfield (IL): Merriam-Webster; 1993. p. 985–6.
[3] Smith EM, Juvinall RC. Mechanics of orthotics. In: Redford JB, editor. Orthotics etcetera. 2nd edition. Baltimore: Williams & Wilkins; 1980. p. 22.
[4] Mizrahi J. Variation of time-distance parameters of the stride as related to clinical gait improvements in hemiplegics. Scand J Rehabil Med 1982;14:133–40.
[5] Valmassy RL. Lower extremity function and normal mechanics. In: Clinical biomechanics of the lower extremities. St. Louis: Mosby; 1996. p. 32–5.
[6] Rasch PJ, Burke RK. Kinesiology and applied anatomy. 3rd edition. Philadelphia: Lea & Febiger; 1967.
[7] Fitts P. Perceptual-motor skills learning. In: Melton A, editor. Categories of human learning. New York: Academic Press; 1964. p. 243.
[8] O'Sullivan SB. Strategies to improve motor control and motor learning. In: O'Sullivan SB, Schmitz TJ, editors. Physical rehabilitation assessment and treatment. 3rd edition. Philadelphia: FA Davis; 1994. p. 237–44.
[9] Daniels L, Williams M, Worthingham C. Introduction. In: Manual muscle testing, techniques of manual examination. 2nd edition. Philadelphia: WB Saunders; 1956, reprinted 1968. p. 1–11.
[10] Kendal FP, McCreary EK. Muscles: testing and function. 2nd edition. Philadelphia: Williams & Wilkins; 1994.
[11] Reese NB, Bandy WD. Joint range of motion and muscle length testing. Philadelphia: WB Saunders; 2002.
[12] Webber D, senior editor. The Canadian Association of Prosthetists and Orthotists: biomechanics and gait. In: Clinical aspects of lower extremity orthotics. Ontario: Elgan Enterprises; 1990. p. 61–81.
[13] Schmitz TJ. Preambulation and gait training. In: O'Sullivan SB, Schmitz TJ, editors. Physical rehabilitation assessment and treatment. 3rd edition. Philadelphia: FA Davis; 1994. p. 251–74.
[14] Knott M, Voss DE. Introduction. In: Proprioceptive neuromuscular facilitation patterns and techniques. 2nd edition. New York: Harper & Row; 1968. p. 9–16.
[15] Williams M, Worthingham C. Principles of treatment and exercises for the various areas: low back area. In: Therapeutic exercise for body alignment and function. Philadelphia: WB Saunders; 1957, reprinted 1966. p. 41–2.
[16] Menezes A. Mental control over physical movement. In: The complete guide to Joseph H. Pilates techniques of physical conditioning. Alameda: Hunter House; 2000. p. 14–29.
[17] Ungaro A. Introduction, the language of Pilates. In: Pilates—body in motion. New York: Dorling Kindersley; 2002. p. 14–21.

[18] Latey P. What is Pilates? In: Modern Pilates. Australia: Allen & Unwin; 2001. p. 15–23.
[19] Clark MA. Pediatric orthoses: bracing in myelomeningoecele. In: Goldberg B, Hsu JD, editors. Atlas of orthoses and assistive devices. 3rd edition. St. Louis: Mosby; 1997. p. 546.
[20] Smith J, Kelly E, Monks J. Introduction to yoga-Pilates. In: Pilates and yoga. London: Hermes House; 2004. p. 134–5.

PHYSICAL MEDICINE
AND REHABILITATION
CLINICS OF
NORTH AMERICA

ELSEVIER
SAUNDERS

Phys Med Rehabil Clin N Am
17 (2006) 245–263

Laser Imaging and Computer-Aided Design and Computer-Aided Manufacture in Prosthetics and Orthotics

John P. Spaeth, MS

Hanger Orthopedic Group, Inc., Two Bethesda Metro Center, Bethesda, MD 20814, USA

Computer-aided design (CAD) and computer-aided manufacture (CAM) have remained in their infancy since the 1970s. Several systems have surfaced touting a solution for the rehabilitation specialist during that time, but they all have fallen short of minimal expectations, and this has resulted in, at best, a minimal embrace of CAD/CAM technology in orthotic and prosthetic rehabilitation. In 2004, the Hanger Orthopedic Group, Inc., formed a technology committee to conduct a landmark investigation into the use of CAD/CAM for orthotists and prosthetists in their daily practice. This investigation produced the following conclusions (JP Spaeth, et al, unpublished online survey, 2004):

1. Electromechanical scanners that merely scan a plaster cast are inaccurate.
2. Contact scanning using a touch or "rub" wand creates soft tissue distortion.
3. A laser or refracted light three-dimensional imaging device is necessary for accurate image capture.
4. The imaging device has to be portable and move easily between clinical environments.
5. The imaging device has to service all orthotic and prosthetic patients so that multiple devices do not need to be employed.
6. Digital images need to become a permanent part of the patient's record.
7. Modification of the images that can be performed directly by the practitioner or a collaborative network need to exist to consult on modifications.

E-mail address: JSpaeth@Hanger.com

1047-9651/06/$ - see front matter © 2006 Elsevier Inc. All rights reserved.
doi:10.1016/j.pmr.2005.11.005

8. All digital information transfer systems have to be compliant with the Health Insurance Portability and Accountability Act (HIPAA).
9. Existing file formats are inadequate to handle multiaxis limb components.
10. Current CAD programs cannot accommodate direct input of all limb component images and cannot handle multiple joints in a single segment.
11. Computer numeric control (CNC) milling machines are not equipped to handle the advanced file formats and cannot carve all limb components.

To the practitioner new to CAD/CAM, the above-summarized analysis may seem esoteric. If that is the case, the practitioner should access the CAD/CAM overview available at www.hanger.com/insignia for a comprehensive look at how digital imaging is used for patient care.

In 2005, the Hanger Orthopedic Group, Inc., developed a digital imaging system called INSIGNIA. This system comprises six technologically advanced state-of-the-art components:

1. Laser imaging wand and motion tracking system
2. CAD software designed specifically to handle multiple limb segments
3. Clinical research and development center for the development of advanced features based on feedback from the users
4. Education center to train more than 600 practitioners in the use of the INSIGNIA laser imaging device and CAD software
5. Establishment of a central design center to collaborate on difficult designs
6. Fabrication services provided by a network of specially designed CNC milling machines

This article discusses each of the six above-listed components in detail. It is hoped that the reader comes to understand the value of the system in his or her practice and uses the system in conjunction with the orthotic and prosthetic rehabilitative care of patients.

INSIGNIA laser imaging components

The first component of the imaging system is an integration of three discrete devices: (1) laser wand, (2) motion tracker, and (3) computer with imaging software (Fig. 1). A cursory examination of the laser imaging equipment reveals that the entire component suite fits into a portable and easily transportable case. The imaging can be performed in many different clinical environments. Virtually any space suitable for patient care can be used to set up the equipment and perform the scan. The only limitations would be an environment that was subject to bright full-spectrum light, as in large windows with streaming sunlight, and an environment that was rich with electromagnetic interference caused by a machine in a nearby location without complete containment.

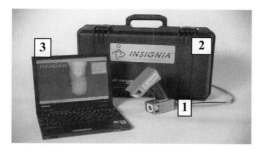

Fig. 1. INSIGNIA laser imaging system components: (1) laser wand, (2) tracking system, and (3) computer with proprietary CAD software. (Courtesy of Hanger Prosthetics & Orthotics; with permission.)

The small size of this equipment and its portable profile allows the orthotic and prosthetic practitioner to take the equipment into the patient's home, nursing home, hospital, rehabilitation center, or physician's office. This scaled-down equipment profile was another innovation of the Hanger INSIGNIA development team. Before this innovation, some of the equipment that was suitable for some patients could not go where the patent was. Many patients who were immobile did not have access to CAD/CAM because the equipment could not be moved.

There are many situations in which the physiatrist might not use CAD/CAM technology because of the lack of portability of the equipment. Postoperative or early intervention prosthetic care now can occur before the patient becomes ambulatory. With INSIGNIA, the early postoperative patient now can be attended bedside with the INSIGNIA laser scanner. One use for this noninvasive procedure is to fit KIWI or NUT-MEGGER (Hanger proprietary postoperative protective/compressive dressings) to the patient, without the patient ever leaving his or her bed (Fig. 2).

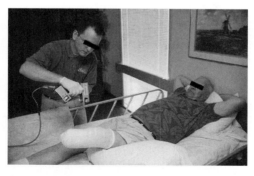

Fig. 2. Patient being imaged for a NUT-MEGGER, which is a protective plastic shell that also maintains an appropriate knee flexion angle. (Courtesy of Hanger Prosthetics & Orthotics; with permission.)

Cranial helmets

The cranial helmet always has presented a unique challenge for orthotists. The age of the child who typically receives this type of service precludes
him or her from following instructions about positioning the cranium. Rapid
head movement, crying, and reaching for the laser wand characterize these
young children. The alternative to laser imaging requires that the child's cranium be wrapped in a messy plaster cast, however, and the practitioner must
try to immobilize the child while the plaster sets. This cranial casting procedure is quite uncomfortable for the child. The INSIGNIA laser image is
captured in less than 2 minutes (typically 1 minute) and is totally noninvasive (Figs. 3 and 4).

Because of the advanced motion tracking ability of the INSIGNIA system, the child's head movement is tracked, which allows the software to
compensate for the movement and correspondingly adjust the image so
that it is distortion-free. Beyond the data acquisition aspect of the INSIG-
NIA scanner, which enhances the patient experience, the system also makes
an empirical analysis of the volumetric and measurement data associated
with cranial dimensioning. The physician receives printed reports that not
only contain the image of the cranium before treatment, but also include
an image of the cranium after treatment. This image becomes part of the
permanent patient record to be recalled on a subsequent visit. In this way,
the physician can determine the efficacy of the treatment and monitor the re-
shaping process closely. Additionally, these images are profiled numerically
so that an actual measurement charting of cranial measurements is created.
Fig. 5 shows a comparative image of the same child before and after
treatment.

Spinal imaging

Several issues concerning spinal orthoses are addressed with INSIGNIA.
Many patients who have experienced spinal trauma cannot stand to be

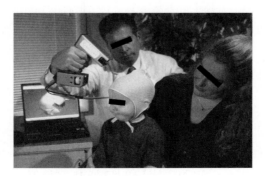

Fig. 3. Laser scan of a 14-month-old infant. (Courtesy of Hanger Prosthetics & Orthotics; with
permission.)

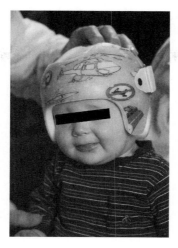

Fig. 4. Infant wearing a Hanger Cranial Band produced directly from the scan performed in Fig. 3. (Courtesy of Hanger Prosthetics & Orthotics; with permission.)

casted for their spinal jacket. The casting procedure is painful and invasive, particularly in a postoperative environment. Typically, the industry has addressed this issue by taking simple tape measurements of the patient and using custom-modified templates to make the actual thoracolumbosacral orthosis (TLSO) body jackets.

The skilled INSIGNIA user can use the laser imaging device while the patient is lying in bed. For symmetric patients (ie, patients whose left topography is approximately equal to their right topography) and patients who have little or no asymmetry to their spine, the patient need only roll to one side,

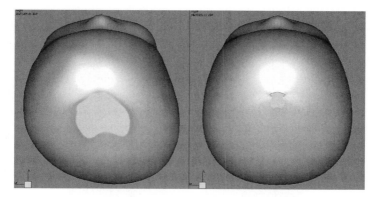

Fig. 5. View of the child's cranium before treatment with a helmet (*left*). Same cranium after 3-month treatment with a Hanger Cranial Band helmet (*right*). The asymmetry is clearly visible on the left. (Courtesy of Hanger Prosthetics & Orthotics; with permission.)

and the scan, which takes approximately 3 minutes, is performed on one side of the torso (Fig. 6). The software builds the opposite side after verifying some basic anatomic measurements taken by the orthotist.

Positioning of the patient often can be achieved by adjusting the head and foot sections of the hospital bed. After the scan of the patient is complete, the hemispherical scan is processed in the Hanger INSIGNIA proprietary software, and a full TLSO is produced (Fig. 7). In addition to the entire procedure being fast and painless to the patient, the physician is provided with a full image of the patient and full set of anatomic measures to be included in the patient's chart as part of the permanent record. The TLSO is sent to the central design center, where it is modified based on the physical characteristics of the patient and the nature of the injury or pathology. The digital design is sent to a fabrication production center, where the actual plastic is molded and final assembly procedures are performed (Fig. 8).

Ankle-foot orthoses

The ankle-foot orthosis is likely one of the most common orthoses applied on a daily basis. Typically, the plaster casting process involves wrapping the entire tibial section of the leg and the ankle and foot circumferentially. After the plaster sets, a cast cutter is used to split the plaster cast down the length of the anterior surface. Because the cast encapsulates the entire lower leg and foot, after the anterior cut is made, the cast must be spread so that the patient can doff the cast. When the cast is spread, it undergoes tremendous distortion.

With the INSIGNIA laser scanner, the patient does not have to endure the casting procedure or the cutting procedure afterward. The leg and foot is simply scanned with the fan of laser light in a matter of minutes (Figs. 9 and 10). There are several advantages of scanning the leg for an ankle-foot orthosis instead of casting. First is the obvious advantage of not exposing the patient or his or her wounds to nonsterile plaster and water. The second advantage is the fine control the orthotist has in making

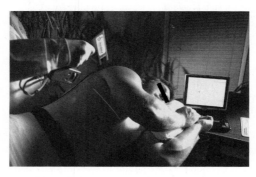

Fig. 6. Patient lies on one side while being scanned for a symmetric TLSO. (Courtesy of Hanger Prosthetics & Orthotics; with permission.)

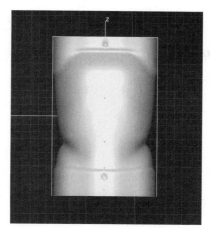

Fig. 7. TLSO shown on CAD computer screen while it is being designed. (Courtesy of Hanger Prosthetics & Orthotics; with permission.)

angular corrections to the foot/ankle. The angular changes made to any of the joints are measured in 1° increments. Regardless of whether the adjustments are rotational or axial in nature, the INSIGNIA proprietary software can make and track the adjustment. Relatively complex changes to plantar flexion or dorsiflexion angles or forefoot changes to varus or valgus can be achieved easily (Figs. 11 and 12). The software tracks and quantifies these changes, which become part of the patient's permanent record.

When a CROW boot (Charcot restraint orthotic walker) is required, the laser scan is used as the basis of the construction of the walker itself (Fig. 13). Often these are accommodative, but are used to unweight the ulcer on the plantar surface of the foot. After the patient's extremity is scanned, weight-bearing areas are created easily on any surface. Conversely, weight-relief areas also are created where necessary. The key concept is that the

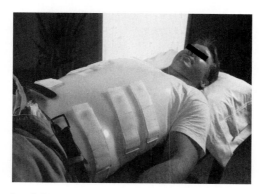

Fig. 8. Patient wearing finished TLSO. (Courtesy of Hanger Prosthetics & Orthotics; with permission.)

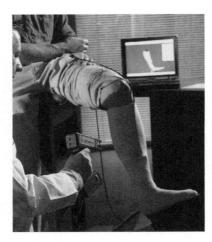

Fig. 9. Patient being scanned for an ankle-foot orthosis. The foot is positioned in as close to neutral as possible before scanning. This ensures the least angular change to the shape in the CAD modification. (Courtesy of Hanger Prosthetics & Orthotics; with permission.)

modification is performed digitally so that any angle changes or pressure areas are recorded and controlled with great accuracy. If a foam liner is required, it too can be made over a scanned model. As the patient's volume decreases, reductions can be made easily in the CAD program, and another smaller liner can be produced.

Pedorthotics and custom shoes

The INSIGNIA scanner has the ability to scan the foot under load conditions also; this is important when tissue displacement on the plantar

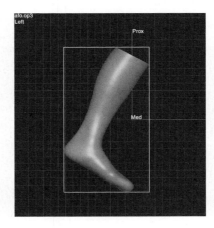

Fig. 10. Scan of a patient's leg ready for modification for an ankle-foot orthosis. (Courtesy of Hanger Prosthetics & Orthotics; with permission.)

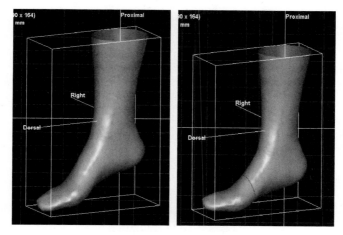

Fig. 11. Unmodified scan with plantar grade deformity (*left*). Same scan with a 15° dorsiflexion correction (*right*). (Courtesy of Hanger Prosthetics & Orthotics; with permission.)

surface of the foot is an issue. The patient is able to stand on a specially treated piece of glass, and the laser can scan through to the plantar surface of the foot. Pedorthotic appliance and custom shoes can be made from a foot scan taken in this way. Existing methods of casting or producing pedorthotics range from looking at an inkblot of the foot, to standing in a foam box and crushing the low-density foam to attempt to transfer the topography of the foot, to hand casting with plaster. Because of the ability of INSIGNIA to scan through special glass, the plantar surface of the foot is accurately detailed with or without weight bearing (Figs. 14 and 15). The

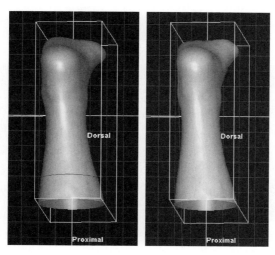

Fig. 12. Unmodified scan showing forefoot valgus (*left*). Same scan showing 15° of forefoot valgus correction (*right*). (Courtesy of Hanger Prosthetics & Orthotics; with permission.)

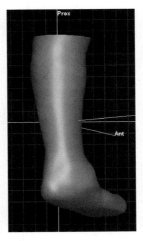

Fig. 13. Scan of a Charcot foot that has been modified and ready to carve for a CROW boot. (Courtesy of Hanger Prosthetics & Orthotics; with permission.)

INSIGNIA laser scan produces a direct conversion to a positive image so that no inaccuracy with image transfer occurs as in traditional methods.

Burn garments and facemasks

Orthotists and prosthetists often are called on to provide facemasks to treat scar tissue from burns or fractures of the face or nose. Traditionally, casting for a facemask required the patient to lie down while a soupy casting solution was poured over the face. The patient had to keep his or her eyes closed and breathe through straws until the casting solution set to a rubber-like substance. The patient's face was immersed in this solution for 15 minutes while the curing process occurred.

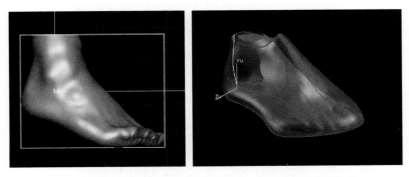

Fig. 14. Image produced by a non–weight-bearing image of the foot (*left*). The foot scan image was corrected and is shown inside a virtual representation of a shoe last (*right*). From here, the shape is carved into a last, around which a custom shoe can be made. (Courtesy of Hanger Prosthetics & Orthotics; with permission.)

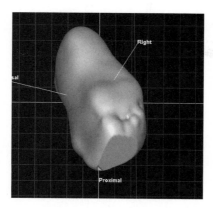

Fig. 15. The foot scan as it appears with no weight bearing. Foot orthotics can be made directly over this shape. (Courtesy of Hanger Prosthetics & Orthotics; with permission.)

The INSIGNIA laser scanner merely fans the laser light over the face and in four or five passes captures the detail of the face or scars on the skin (Fig. 16). After the patient is scanned, a positive of the face is carved out of a special material, which allows for modification by the treating therapist after the mask is made (Figs. 17 and 18). Often the therapist may want to apply more or less pressure to a specific area as the therapy progresses. The special carved material allows for this process to occur. Many of these incremental adjustments can be made without having to remake the mask.

Athletic/fracture facemasks are fabricated in the same way. The fit for an athletic mask is not nearly as crucial, and, typically, incremental adjustments do not need to be made after the patient begins wearing the mask. Typically, athletic masks require a much less involved trim line, and so more of the face is unencumbered by the device.

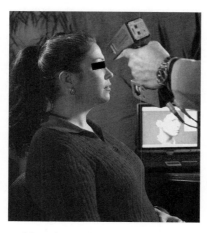

Fig. 16. Patient being scanned for a facemask with the INSIGNIA scanner. (Courtesy of Hanger Prosthetics & Orthotics; with permission.)

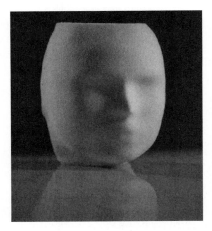

Fig. 17. Facemask positive carved from special material that allows modifications. (Courtesy of Hanger Prosthetics & Orthotics; with permission.)

Burn garment measuring

Because of the accuracy of the INSIGNIA laser scanner, all of the images can be used where detailed measurements are required. One of the most intriguing uses for the detailed measuring capability of INSIGNIA is to employ the image for measuring patients for various compression garments. Traditionally, the patient must be measured with a tape measure every half inch or so along an axis. This is a time-consuming task for the clinician and an arduous task for the patient, especially when one considers the traumatic and painful cause of the scarring. With the INSIGNIA laser scanner, the patient is asked to stand in an anatomically neutral position, and the

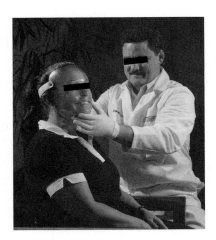

Fig. 18. Patient being fitted with the clear facemask made from the carved model in Fig. 17. (Courtesy of Hanger Prosthetics & Orthotics; with permission.)

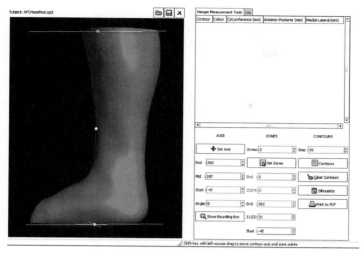

Fig. 19. Lower extremity scan ready to have measurement analysis performed by INSIGNIA software. (Courtesy of Hanger Prosthetics & Orthotics; with permission.)

affected body part is scanned (Figs. 19 and 20). If the patient cannot stand, accommodations usually can be made for the patient to sit or lie down for most measurements.

The measurement software also can be used for many types of volumetric analyses. Current research is under way for volume measurements regarding lymph edema. In this case, the scan would be taken, and linear measurements along with volumetric information would be recorded. At the next

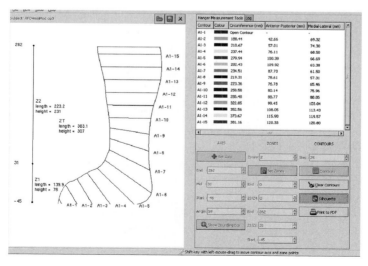

Fig. 20. Lower extremity scan silhouetted, and dimensioned ready for garment fabrication. (Courtesy of Hanger Prosthetics & Orthotics; with permission.)

clinic visit, the patient would be rescanned and dimensioned as described previously. At that point, the two scans could be compared, and a quick and accurate assessment of volume change would be rendered.

Because the INSIGNIA scanner can measure negative surface equally well, an ulcerated area can be scanned, and a volumetric analysis can be performed. At a subsequent clinic visit, the wound is rescanned, and a volumetric analysis via a comparison of the two scans is rendered. The wound care specialist can see at a glance whether the wound has decreased in volume since the last visit.

Prosthetic laser scanner applications

Most prosthetic scans are cylindrical in shape, which makes them prime candidates for the old .AOP file format. This is the format that the American Academy of Orthotists and Prosthetists created years ago when prosthetic CAD/CAM was in its infancy. Although the shapes are basically cylindrical, many prosthetic patients present with irregular shapes ranging from bulbous to extreme bony prominence. INSIGNIA is able to capture and modify all prosthetic shapes effectively. Of particular interest is the scanning of upper extremity patients. With the highly involved shoulder disarticulation patient, to place relief and pressure areas exactly and determine electrode placement, the patient often was subjected to two or more check socket fittings. With the INSIGNIA scan, the same patient can be fitted routinely with one or two check socket fittings (Fig. 21).

High-level upper extremity amputees also benefit from the fact that INSIGNIA can carve the entire upper torso. The socket and harnessing/

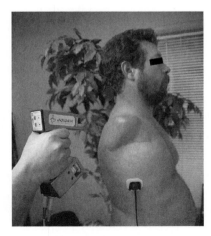

Fig. 21. Shoulder disarticulation patient being scanned for a check socket. The motion sensor is attached to the patient's body to track any movement during the scan. (Courtesy of Hanger Prosthetics & Orthotics; with permission.)

suspension components can be molded to an exact replica of the patient as if the hot plastic were actually being applied to the patient for molding (Fig. 22).

Other prosthetic scans also are beneficial and less invasive than plaster casting. In the case of a bulbous shape, the residual limb is wrapped in plaster. Because of the bulbous distal end, there is no way to remove the cast but to cut it off. This results in distortions and an uncomfortable experience for the patient. With INSIGNIA, the shape is captured in seconds with no distortion and extreme accuracy of $\pm$ 1 mm. Because of the portability of the INSIGNIA system, the scanner can be moved around the patient, and irregular shapes can be captured even if they do not fit into a gantry-type mounted scanning device. This makes the INSIGNIA laser suitable not only for transtibial and transfemoral amputations, but also Symes, Chopart, and hip disarticulation (Figs. 23–26).

Summary

Although Hanger Orthopedic Group, Inc., has been developing clinical protocols for its INSIGNIA scanner for more than 2 years, there are many applications that are currently in development and will be released over the next 2-year period after this publication. It is the goal of Hanger Orthopedic Group, Inc., to replace all plaster casting procedures with the laser scan and move toward a paperless environment where all images and documents are passed through its virtual network. INSIGNIA currently has five major production centers throughout the United States, which support more than 600 INSIGNIA certified clinicians. These clinicians staff

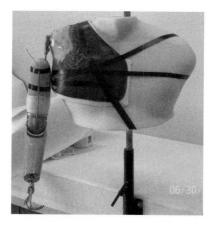

Fig. 22. The entire upper torso of the patient can be scanned and carved so that the clinician can build the prosthesis around the carving as if he or she were building it with the patient trying it on at every step. (Courtesy of Hanger Prosthetics & Orthotics; with permission.)

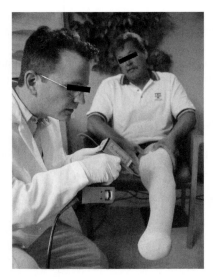

Fig. 23. Typical Symes amputation being scanned. (Courtesy of Hanger Prosthetics & Orthotics; with permission.)

more than 600 clinics in North America, all under the Hanger company name. The central fabrication service and the central design center processes hundreds of shapes per day (Fig. 27).

So that any clinician in the field can use the expertise of the central designers and central fabricators to help with overflow or problems they might be having, the network that exists within Hanger is tied together and enhanced by INSIGNIA. Through virtual modification and centralization of

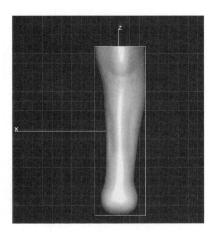

Fig. 24. The Symes scan as it looks in the INSIGNIA CAD program modified and ready to carve. (Courtesy of Hanger Prosthetics & Orthotics; with permission.)

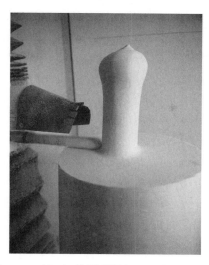

Fig. 25. Symes shape being carved in the INSIGNIA carver from a block of foam. (Courtesy of Hanger Prosthetics & Orthotics; with permission.)

these services, each patient receives the virtual collaboration of several clinicians with a total of years of experience. INSIGNIA has enhanced the patient experience. The enhancement is not only in removing the plaster from the process, but also in exposing each patient to the team of prosthetic experts working collaboratively behind the scenes.

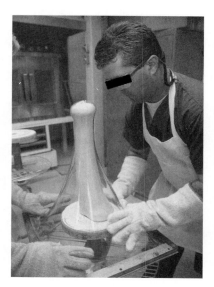

Fig. 26. After the shape is carved, a negative socket is made by pulling a piece of hot plastic over it and vacuum forming it. (Courtesy of Hanger Prosthetics & Orthotics; with permission.)

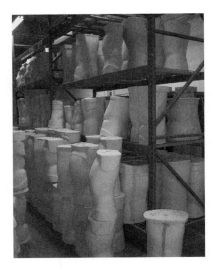

Fig. 27. Shapes that have been carved at one of the central production centers. (Courtesy of Hanger Prosthetics & Orthotics; with permission.)

The rehabilitation industry continues to be bombarded with compliance paperwork and justifications. The INSIGNIA scan and resulting measurement reports give inherent strength to justifications based on volume change, surgical revisions, or tissue change. The files are kept in a data warehouse where they are vaulted and preserved presumably forever. Also, any of the shape graphics or measurement instruments can be printed into a discrete report that can become part of the patient's permanent record. Many physicians receive update letters from their orthotic and prosthetic clinician with a status update before and after treatment of their patient. This update includes a descriptive narrative, a printout of the pertinent metrics, a printout of the scan graphic, and often a digital image of the patient wearing the device (Fig. 28).

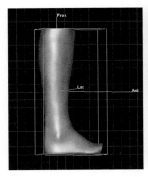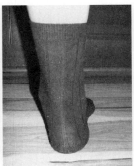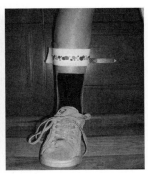

Fig. 28. Typical of a graphic sent to physician for follow-up. Scan of patient (*left*), digital picture showing uncorrected stance (*center*), and patient after receiving orthosis (*right*). (Courtesy of Hanger Prosthetics & Orthotics; with permission.)

The network is HIPAA compliant, and all private health information is held in tight security. If a practitioner does not have a HIPAA agreement in place with Hanger Orthopedic Group, Inc., and would like one, or if a practitioner would like to have an INSIGNIA representative call or visit with more information, the practitioner is encouraged to call 1-800-4-HANGER and request an INSIGNIA in-service or visit INSIGNIA on the web at www.hanger.com.

ELSEVIER
SAUNDERS

Phys Med Rehabil Clin N Am
17 (2006) 265–274

PHYSICAL MEDICINE
AND REHABILITATION
CLINICS OF
NORTH AMERICA

Index

Note: Page numbers of article titles are in **boldface** type.

1047-9651/06/$ - see front matter © 2006 Elsevier Inc. All rights reserved.
doi:10.1016/S1047-9651(06)00012-X

This volume may circulate for 1 week.

Renewals may be made in person or by phone: X6-6050; from outside dial 746-6050. No VMX renewals please. Fines are charged for overdue items. Please renew promptly. Thank you.

Date Due	Date Returned
MAY 2 0 2009	